EAT
TO STAY
YOUNG

EAT
TO STAY
YOUNG

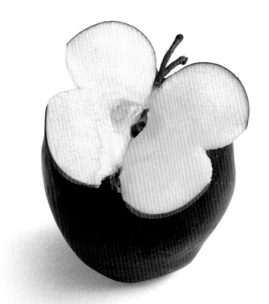

INGREDIENTS & RECIPES
TO REJUVENATE YOUR BODY & MIND

GILL PAUL
NUTRITIONIST: KAREN SULLIVAN, ASET, VTCT, BSC

hamlyn

An Hachette UK Company
www.hachette.co.uk

First published in Great Britain in 2016 by Hamlyn,
a division of Octopus Publishing Group Ltd
Carmelite House
50 Victoria Embankment
London EC4Y 0DZ
www.octopusbooks.co.uk

ISBN 978-0-600-63029-6

A CIP catalogue record for this book
is available from the British Library.

Printed and bound in China

10 9 8 7 6 5 4 3 2 1

All reasonable care has been taken in the preparation
of this book but the information it contains is not
intended to take the place of treatment by a qualified
medical practitioner.

People with known nut allergies should avoid recipes
containing nuts or nut derivatives, and vulnerable
people should avoid dishes containing raw or lightly
cooked eggs.

Both metric and imperial measurements have been
given in all recipes. Use one set of measurements only,
and not a mixture of both.

Standard level spoon measurements
are used in all recipes
1 tablespoon = 15 ml spoon
1 teaspoon = 5 ml spoon

Ovens should be preheated to the specified
temperature – if using a fan-assisted oven,
follow the manufacturer's instructions for adjusting
the time and temperature.

Medium eggs should be used unless otherwise stated.

Some of the recipes in this book have previously
appeared in other titles published by Hamlyn.

Art Director: Jonathan Christie
**Photographic Art Direction, Prop Styling
and Design:** Isabel de Cordova
Photography: Will Heap
Food Styling: Annie Nichols
Assistant Editor: Meri Pentikäinen
Picture Library Manager: Jen Veall
Assistant Production Manager: Caroline Alberti

CONTENTS

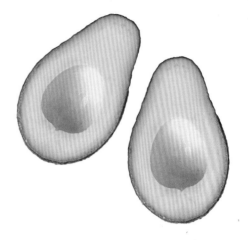

INTRODUCTION

There are lots of anti-ageing treatments, each more extreme than the other, on offer for those who are desperate enough to try them: bee sting and snake venom facials, covering yourself in leeches to detoxify the blood, bull-sperm applications for thinning hair and umpteen surgical procedures to lift, tuck and rearrange your face and body.

However, it's only common sense that the most effective way to slow the ageing process is to treat the cells from within, giving them the nutrients they need to maintain their youthful functions – and the best way to do that is through the food we eat.

How we age

The organs, bones and other tissues in our bodies go through a number of changes as we age. Cells begin to die more frequently and the mechanisms to replace them don't work as efficiently as they used to when we were younger.

Free radicals, the natural waste products of the process by which oxygen from the air we breathe and glucose from our food are used to produce energy, are one of the major causes of ageing. In most young people, free radicals are quickly mopped up and disposed of but, as we age, they are not dealt with so readily and an unhealthy lifestyle creates many more, which can kill off healthy cells or cause them to mutate into cancerous ones.

The rate at which we age

Part of what affects the individual rate at which we age is genetic – our predisposition to disease and the outward signs of ageing come from our parents.

Part is simply due to the amount of wear and tear our bodies receive over time. But a significant part of how well we weather the ageing process is determined by the way we live our lives.

A poor diet, too much alcohol, sunbathing, smoking, stress, pollution: all of these factors hasten the degeneration of tissues in our bodies. A balanced diet that is packed full of delicious anti-ageing nutrients combined with a healthy lifestyle, on the other hand, will keep your body biologically younger for longer.

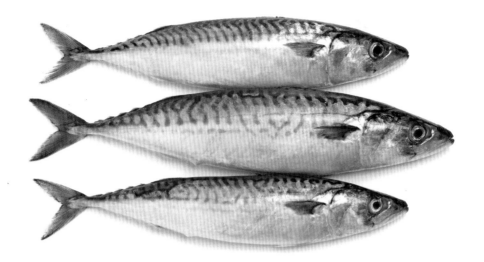

Your weight in middle age

- It's easy for excess weight to creep up as the metabolism slows in middle age, particularly for people with sedentary lifestyles. Those who are plump tend to get fewer wrinkles than their lighter friends because there is a thicker layer of fat under the skin. However, there the advantages end because the strain inflicted on the heart and circulatory system, bones and joints, is likely to give those who are overweight more health problems overall.

- Weight-loss diets in your 40s or 50s can be very ageing, both externally, with wrinkles and pouches of loose skin seemingly appearing overnight, and internally as bones, muscles and organs are leached of nutrients. The solution lies in eating a balanced diet containing all the anti-ageing super-foods, and leading an active life, with at least an hour of exercise a day. Aim to include both aerobic exercise (the kind that makes you out of breath, like running) and muscle-strengthening exercise (such as yoga, t'ai chi or Pilates).

How to eat to stay young

1. Choose whole foods!

Some modern processing methods remove a lot of the goodness from our foods and then replace it with sugars, preservatives and chemical additives. The most important rule for eating to look and feel younger is to buy natural, whole ingredients and cook or prepare them from scratch. That way you will be getting optimum benefits from every last mouthful.

2. Appreciate antioxidants

Foods containing the antioxidant vitamins A, C and E, the mineral selenium and a range of phytonutrients such as lycopene are the front-line defence against free radicals and form a core part of the *Eat to Stay Young* diet. All fruits and vegetables contain useful antioxidants and you should aim for a wide range of different types. A key tip is that the brighter the colours and the fresher they are, the better they'll do their job.

3. Opt for omegas

Omega-3 fatty acids come with several anti-ageing benefits. They help to keep blood cholesterol levels healthy, preventing heart disease; they keep joints supple and prevent inflammation; they keep our brains agile, preventing memory loss; and are nature's own moisturizer for skin and hair. You'll find them in oily fish (sardines, salmon, mackerel and tuna are good sources), as well as nuts, seeds and olive oil.

4. Fill up with fibre

Our digestive systems can slow down as we age, leading to constipation and inefficient absorption of nutrients. Eating plenty of insoluble fibre (found in whole grains and vegetables) adds bulk to food waste and helps to speed its passage. Always choose unrefined carbs such as those in brown rice, wholegrain bread and cereals.

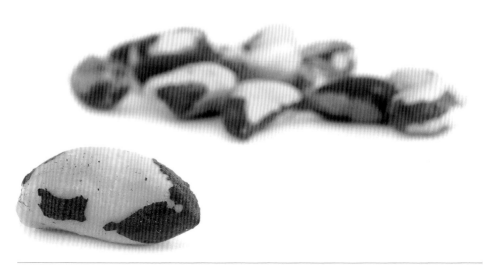

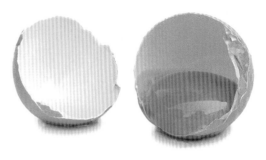

Soluble fibre is also important as it forms a kind of gel with water in the gut and slows down the absorption of sugars into the blood, so it makes us feel full for longer and prevents blood sugar fluctuations. The best sources of soluble fibre include oats, lentils, carrots and all kinds of berries.

5. Keep your bones strong

Making sure you get a good night's sleep makes everything look better the next day, and it is also vital for maintaining healthy blood pressure, balancing mood, regulating hormones, keeping a strong immune system and improving energy levels. Magnesium, calcium and certain amino acids aid restful sleep and you'll find them in abundance in the recipes in this book.

6. Choose B vitamins

B vitamins support the nervous system and help us to relax and cope with stress, as well as maintaining a good metabolic rate and keeping energy levels up. B6 helps with mood and stops premature greying, while B12 helps to stop shrinkage of the brain. Including sources of protein in your diet is essential for providing B vitamins: lean meats, poultry, fish, eggs, beans and pulses and dairy products are all great for protein.

7. Cut the bad habits

You may have got away with puffing on cigarettes, supping cocktails, sunbathing and living on takeaways in your 20s, but the damage will mount as the years go by and no miracle creams will be able to undo it.

Getting started

For many, the biggest change may be to start cooking from scratch. It takes a little longer to cook from raw ingredients but the recipes in this book are not complicated and many can be thrown together in less than 10 minutes. It could be the wisest investment of time you ever make – and you'll find your food bills shrink when you're not paying for fancy packaging and glitzy marketing campaigns anymore.

For all-round good health, and to look and feel younger on every level, just follow the two-week meal planner on pages 30–33. To address specific symptoms of ageing, such as wrinkles or thinning hair, see the problem solver on pages 26–29. On pages 12–25 you will find a list of the powerhouse anti-ageing superfoods along with a host of ways you can introduce them to your regular diet. Try them all, and drink lots of water throughout the day to keep your system well hydrated.

At the age of 20, we have the health and appearance we inherited; at 50 and beyond, we have the face and body we created through our own life choices. Be sure you make wise choices and, while you may not be able to turn back the clock, you can look and feel as though you have.

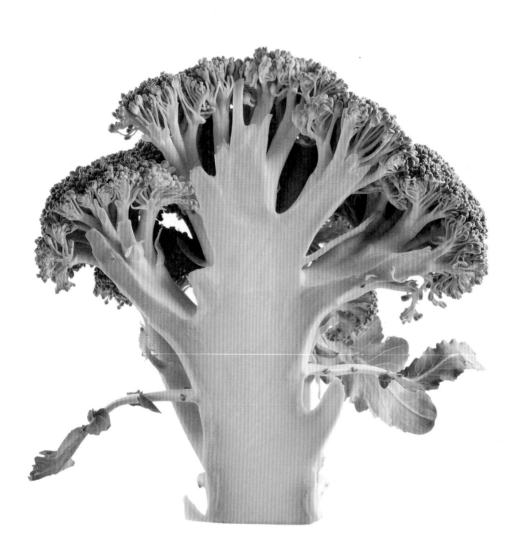

YOUNG
SUPERFOODS

SUPERFOODS

Eaten regularly, these multi-functional foods will have noticeable rejuvenating effects on the whole body, both inside and out.

Brazil nuts

- ✔ Raise energy levels and lift mood
- ✔ Improve memory
- ✔ Encourage healthy skin, hair and nails
- ✔ Promote heart health
- ✔ Reduce degenerative effects of ageing
- ✔ Aid virility and libido
- ✔ Increase metabolism

Rich in healthy fats, brazil nuts are full of selenium, an antioxidant mineral. They also have chemicals that reduce inflammation, slowing down age-related degeneration.

They are rich in...

- → Selenium which balances mood and slows down skin and hair ageing, repairs cell damage, improves elasticity
- → Vitamin E for healthy skin and hair, lower cholesterol and reduced risk of heart attack and stroke
- → Zinc, needed for memory, virility and collagen formation in the skin and joints
- → B vitamins which enhance metabolism, mood, energy, heart health, skin and hair health, and lower cholesterol levels

Use in... salads with feta cheese, grapes and mixed leaves; dip into dark chocolate; grind with fresh tarragon, Parmesan cheese and olive oil for pesto; crumble toppings; muesli; chop finely and scatter over squash or carrot soups; puréed in fresh fruit and yogurt smoothies.

SEE: FRUIT & NUT MUESLI, P42; BERRY & BRAZIL NUT SMOOTHIE, P39; SPICY BRAZIL NUTS, P56.

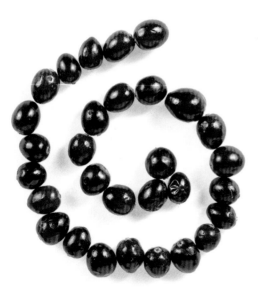

Cranberries

✔ Prevent tooth decay and gum disease
✔ Protect against heart disease
✔ Improve short-term memory
✔ Reduce inflammation and cellulite
✔ Encourage brain and digestive health
✔ Balance blood sugar

Rich in antioxidants which slow down the effects of ageing, and improve heart and dental health, cranberries also aid short-term memory and reduce urinary tract infections. Highly fibrous, they regulate nutrient absorption, digestion and blood sugar.

They are rich in...

→ Proanthocyanidins (PACs) which prevent bacteria from sticking to the surface of teeth and gums (and the urinary tract), reducing the risk of infection and decay
→ Flavonoids to help prevent heart disease, including atherosclerosis, reduce signs of ageing and ease muscle and joint pain
→ Phytonutrients which protect the heart, teeth and gums, reduce high blood pressure and prevent stomach ulcers
→ Vitamins A and C which moisturize the skin, promote collagen, fight free radicals which can cause wrinkles and environmental damage to the skin
→ Chemicals that prevent stomach ulcers

Use in... smoothies; tagines or other chicken, turkey or pork dishes; chutneys; porridge or muesli; snack with nuts and seeds; stuffings; flapjacks, crumbles or muffins; couscous; dried in a salad with green leaves and goats' cheese; juice; baked apple stuffing with almonds, cinnamon and brown sugar.

SEE: CRANBERRY MUFFINS, P69; SPICED RAISIN & CRANBERRY COOKIES, P64; BROCCOLI SALAD WITH DILL & PINE NUTS, P76; CRANBERRY ICE CREAM WITH DARK CHOCOLATE, P118.

Tuna

✔ Improves heart health
✔ Lifts mood and beats fatigue
✔ Lowers blood pressure and cholesterol
✔ Balances blood sugar
✔ Promotes healing and repair of cells
✔ Lowers risk of dementia and aids memory
✔ Keeps joints supple
✔ Improves skin and hair quality
✔ Protects eyesight

The omega-3 oils in tuna help to prevent the degeneration of cells from hair, skin and nails to brain, joints and heart. Tuna is rich in cell-renewing proteins, as well as nutrients that lower cholesterol and blood pressure, and even ensure a good night's sleep.

It's rich in...

→ Selenium which protects the body from free radical damage and helps to support healthy liver and brain function
→ Omega-3 oils for heart and brain health, better memory and mood, reduced inflammation and lower risk of obesity and macular degeneration
→ B vitamins for improved sleep, and red blood cell health to increase energy, and lower risk of atherosclerosis
→ Vitamin D to build and maintain strong bones and teeth, and prevent diabetes

Use in... salad Niçoise; grill tuna kebabs with a citrus marinade; brown rice salad with peppers, spring onions, chopped tomatoes and chickpeas; on jacket potatoes or toasted rye bread with fat-free Greek yogurt, fresh dill and black beans; sushi; form into burgers; grilled on a wholegrain bun; spread with coriander or pesto and roast until just cooked.

SEE: TOASTED QUINOA, TUNA & LENTIL SALAD, P98; SESAME-CRUSTED TUNA WITH GINGER DRESSING, P102; TUNA WITH PEPPERS & FENNEL GRATIN, P104.

Aubergines

✔ Encourage heart and eye health
✔ Balance blood sugar
✔ Lower blood pressure and cholesterol
✔ Enhance memory
✔ Promote healthy digestion
✔ Encourage stronger, healthier hair
✔ Ease fatigue
✔ Help angina
✔ Discourage cellulite

Aubergines are low in calories, high in fibre and bursting with nutrients, such as vitamins A, B and C, which are essential for great skin, hair, eyesight and mood. They also contain potassium, magnesium, phosphorus and calcium, which aid bone and brain health.

They are rich in...

→ Nasunin which protects the fats in brain cells for optimum brain function and helps produce collagen in the skin
→ Chlorogenic acid which reduces bad cholesterol, improves circulation, slows down the degenerative effects of ageing and aids heart health
→ Fibre to balance blood sugar, promote digestion, discourage cellulite and help to protect against type-2 diabetes
→ Potassium to lower blood pressure, ease angina, raise energy levels and lift mood

Use in... vegetable curries; ratatouille; brush slices with olive oil, pepper and basil and grill; roast whole and purée the flesh with lemon juice, salt, cumin and a little live yogurt as a dip or spread for flatbreads or toast; thinly sliced instead of pasta in lasagne; stuff with ricotta cheese, mint, oregano and spinach.

SEE: SMOKY AUBERGINE DIP, P53; AUBERGINE & SESAME NOODLE SALAD, P70; MISO AUBERGINES WITH RICE NOODLES, P100; AUBERGINE, CHICKPEA & PANEER CURRY, P110.

Olive oil

✔ Lowers cholesterol and blood pressure
✔ Promotes brain health
✔ Reduces wrinkles and improves skin
✔ Protects against memory loss and cognitive decline
✔ Supports cardiovascular and bone health
✔ Lifts mood relieves pain
✔ Helps prevent obesity

Olive oil protects against cardiovascular disease and lowers the risk of stroke and heart attacks, while its anti-inflammatory properties reduce pain, support the joints and slow down age-related degeneration. It's rich in antioxidants and studies have also found that it protects against osteoporosis.

It's rich in...

→ Polyphenols, antioxidants which help prevent age-related disease and degeneration, and reduce inflammation
→ Monounsaturated fats which reduce the risk of heart disease and promote skin health (including a reduction in wrinkles), act as anti-inflammatories and prevent cognitive decline
→ Vitamin E which improves the texture and elasticity of the skin, and acts as an antioxidant to protect the body from free radicals
→ Vitamin K for a healthy nervous system, brain function, strong bones and teeth

Use in... stir-fries; drizzle over toast in place of butter or margarine; salad dressing with fresh and dried herbs and lemon juice; bake into crisp, herby flatbreads or biscotti; as the basis for sweet polenta or pistachio cakes; to flavour steamed vegetables and pastas; instead of butter in pastry.

SEE: VIRTUALLY EVERY SALAD DRESSING AND COOKED SAVOURY DISH IN THIS BOOK.

Red peppers

✔ Promote healthy eyesight
✔ Make skin more elastic
✔ Speed up the metabolism
✔ Encourage heart health
✔ Lower blood pressure
✔ Aid digestion
✔ Lower cholesterol

With a wide range of nutrients to encourage health and wellbeing on every level, red peppers are rich in vitamin C which is vital for hair health, eyesight, energy levels, skin, nails and joints. They also contain silicon to improve the condition of hair and nails, and magnesium and vitamin B6 to enhance mood, relaxation, healthy sleep patterns and combat premature greying. Peppers are also full of antioxidants to help delay the signs of ageing.

They are rich in...

→ Lycopene which encourages elasticity in the skin and stimulates collagen production, while supporting healthy heart function
→ Vitamin A which supports healthy eyesight and lutein which lowers the risk of macular degeneration and cataracts
→ Potassium to lower blood pressure, prevent angina, encourage the health of the brain and nervous system, and raise mood
→ Vitamin C, an excellent antioxidant which also supports the health of skin and joints, and prevents premature greying

Use in... ratatouille with aubergines, courgettes and tomatoes; stuff with herby brown rice and feta cheese and roast; slice and eat raw with hummus or other dips; roast and serve in sandwiches with hummus or haloumi; slice and add to quiches, omelettes or scrambled eggs; roast and purée with herbs for a delicious pasta or pizza sauce.

SEE: BROCCOLI & RED PEPPER FRITTATA, P46; MEDITERRANEAN STUFFED PEPPERS, P82; TUNA WITH PEPPERS & FENNEL GRATIN, P104; HEARTY RATATOUILLE, P108.

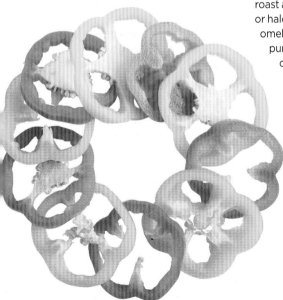

Tomatoes

✔ Protect the skin and bones
✔ Reduce the risk of cancers, arthritis and joint problems
✔ Lower cholesterol
✔ Encourage heart health and eyesight

Tomatoes will provide you with a burst of vitamins, minerals and other elements which promote the faster growth of new cells – including cells in the skin.

They are rich in...
→ Lycopene which protects the skin from sunburn and UV rays and promotes the formation and renewal of collagen; also important to protect against cancer, heart disease and osteoporosis
→ Phytonutrients which lower cholesterol and prevent atherosclerosis
→ Vitamin C for the production of collagen required for healthy hair and skin; it also reduces the risk of arthritis, macular degeneration and joint problems
→ Biotin which is necessary for healthy skin and hair, and critical for cell turnover and heart health; adequate amounts in the diet can prevent premature greying of hair

Use in... pasta sauces; casseroles, stews and soups; roast and top with oregano, olive oil and a sprinkling of pecorino; sun-dried in sandwiches and salads; topping for bruschetta, baked feta or foil-cooked white fish; salad with red onions and basil; cherry tomatoes as a snack; juices with celery salt and lemon.

SEE: HUEVOS RANCHEROS, P48; BROCCOLI & RED PEPPER FRITTATA, P46; MEDITERRANEAN STUFFED PEPPERS, P82; AVOCADO & TOMATO TOSTADOS, P60; BRUSCHETTA WITH TOMATOES & BASIL, P62; GAZPACHO, P83; HEARTY RATATOUILLE, P108.

Pomegranates

✔ Encourage healthy digestion and elimination
✔ Balance weight and blood sugar
✔ Lift mood
✔ Regulate blood pressure
✔ Preserve collagen in skin
✔ Promote heart and eye health
✔ Lower cholesterol
✔ Regenerate cartilage in joints
✔ Prevent hair loss

Pomegranate seeds and the bitter white pith contain key antioxidants to reverse signs of ageing. They also increase oxygen levels to the heart, encourage moist, supple skin, aid symptoms of inflammatory conditions such as arthritis and strengthen hair follicles, preventing loss of hair.

They are rich in...
→ Fibre to balance weight and blood sugar levels, promote digestion and ease constipation
→ Folic acid for a healthy nervous system and reduced inflammation
→ Punicalagin which lowers blood pressure and cholesterol, and reduces the risk of angina and atherosclerosis
→ Vitamin K and manganese for bone health

Use in... fresh, fruity salsas served with tagines, pork or lamb dishes; smoothies with berries and live yogurt; breakfast cereals and muesli; on top of quartered pears with goats' cheese; nutty wild rice or quinoa salads; the juice to glaze ribs, sprinkled with the seeds.

SEE: BLUEBERRY POMEGRANATE SMOOTHIE, P36; FRUIT SALSA & CINNAMON CRISPS, P114; CARROT & BEETROOT TABBOULEH, P78; BROCCOLI SALAD WITH DILL & PINE NUTS, P76; GUAVA-GLAZED PORK TENDERLOIN, P96; POMEGRANATE PANNA COTTA, P122.

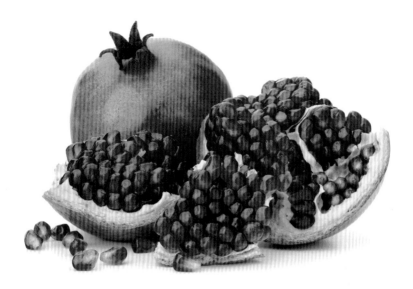

Watercress

✔ Prevents bone loss
✔ Lowers blood pressure
✔ Stabilizes heart rate
✔ Supports health of skin and hair
✔ Required for cardiovascular health
✔ Boosts libido
✔ Fights fatigue
✔ Encourages healthy gums
✔ Enhances digestion

With more calcium than milk, more vitamin C than most fruits and plenty of iron, this peppery vegetable improves digestive function, boosts energy levels, encourages healthy eyesight and has been used across the centuries to improve libido. It's also high in fibre which can balance blood sugar levels and improve digestion.

It's rich in...
➔ Vitamin K which can help to prevent memory loss and encourage the health of bones and teeth

➔ Vitamin C for healthy skin, hair, connective tissues and gums, as well as improving immunity
➔ Vitamin A for healthy skin and eyes, reducing the risk of macular degeneration and cataracts, as well as preventing night blindness
➔ Flavonoids such as lutein, zeaxanthin and carotene which promote vision and cardiovascular health

Use in... sandwiches instead of lettuce; in salads with avocado; braise with garlic and lemon; use instead of spinach in stuffed pasta dishes; blend with apples for a nourishing smoothie; use as a base for pesto instead of basil; simmer with leeks and stock then purée for a light soup; add to lightly cooked omelettes or frittatas with goats' cheese.

SEE: WATERCRESS SOUP WITH CHEESY OATCAKES, P88; BROCCOLI SALAD WITH DILL & PINE NUTS, P76.

Carrots

- ✔ Boost liver function
- ✔ Ease constipation
- ✔ Lower cholesterol
- ✔ Support heart and bone health
- ✔ Boost immunity and metabolism
- ✔ Promote healthy eyesight
- ✔ Reduce wrinkles, age spots and dry skin
- ✔ Promote strong, healthy hair
- ✔ Raise libido

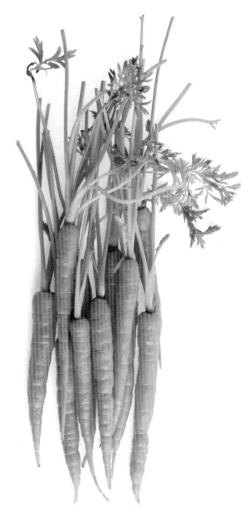

Carrots stimulate liver function which helps digestion, hormone balance and energy levels. They are high in fibre to help elimination and full of nutrients that prevent bloating.

They are rich in...
- → Fibre which lowers cholesterol, balances blood sugar and aids healthy digestion
- → Vitamins C and E to aid circulation to the scalp, which encourages hair growth and prevents premature greying
- → Antioxidants and polyacetylenes to protect the heart
- → Beta-carotene which improves skin, heart and liver health, and converts in the retina to rhodopsin, needed for night vision and prevention of cataracts and macular degeneration
- → Vitamin K for a healthy nervous system, bone health and brain function

Use in... stews; casseroles; soups; juices; salads; raw with guacamole, hummus or other dips; roast with thyme, lemon and a little olive oil; soup with orange rind; grated, add to any cakes and scones; roast and add to sandwiches and wraps.

SEE: CARROT & LENTIL MUFFINS, P66; CARROT CRISPS WITH HONEY YOGURT DIP, P58; CARROT, CORIANDER & LENTIL SOUP, P91; CARROT & BEETROOT TABBOULEH, P78; CARROT & PUY LENTIL SALAD, P75.

Fennel

- ✔ Improves digestion and eases constipation
- ✔ Lowers cholesterol and blood pressure
- ✔ Enhances brain function
- ✔ Protects eyesight
- ✔ Encourages heart health
- ✔ Prevents inflammation
- ✔ Balances mood
- ✔ Improves hair and skin
- ✔ Discourages cellulite

Fennel is a versatile vegetable which can be prepared in a wide variety of ways. It is a treasure trove of nutrients and even half a bulb will supply good levels of vitamins A, B and C, fibre, potassium, folic acid, manganese, phosphorus, calcium, iron and copper.

It's rich in...
→ Iron and histidine which encourage the supply of oxygenated blood throughout the body, improving brain, heart, skin and hair health
→ Antioxidants, such as vitamin C and the amino acid arginine, which prevent macular degeneration and other age-related eye problems
→ Potassium which facilitates connections within the brain and also lowers blood pressure and the risk of angina, raises energy levels, lifts mood and regulates the heartbeat
→ Fibre to balance blood sugar levels, promote healthy digestion and assimilation of nutrients and prevent constipation, while discouraging cellulite
→ Sulphur and amino acids to encourage healthy hair and skin

Use in... stews, soups and casseroles; slice thinly in salads or serve as a crudité with dips; roast with a medley of other vegetables in a little olive oil, lemon juice and black pepper; steam, braise or sauté as an accompaniment; juice with apples or carrots; roast and purée with potatoes or other root vegetables.

SEE: CITRUS OLIVES, P50; FENNEL & CUMIN WALDORF SALAD, P74; FENNEL & MUSHROOM TARTS, P86; CARAMELIZED GARLIC TART, P106; HEARTY RATATOUILLE, P108; FENNEL-ROASTED LAMB WITH FIGS, P94; TUNA WITH PEPPERS & FENNEL GRATIN, P104.

Oats

✔ Nourish the nervous system
✔ Balance blood sugar levels
✔ Enhance memory and energy levels
✔ Encourage healthy digestion
✔ Promote restful sleep
✔ Lower cholesterol and blood pressure
✔ Lift mood, energy and libido

Rich in vitamins, fibre and a wealth of other nutrients such as healthy fatty acids and protein, oats are particularly beneficial for their impact on the brain and digestion.

They are rich in...
→ Zinc which is needed for immunity, libido, energy levels, memory and collagen formation in the skin and joints
→ B vitamins to encourage the health of the nervous system, aid restful sleep, balance mood and encourage healthy skin and hair
→ Soluble and insoluble fibre to improve digestive health and the absorption of nutrients from food, and to balance blood sugar and cholesterol
→ Avenanthramides, antioxidants which help to prevent cardiovascular disease

Use in... porridge, homemade muesli and baked breakfast goods; use as a topping for crumbles and sweet and savoury pies; enjoy in oat bars and biscuits as healthy snacks; use as a coating for baked fish or chicken; use in homemade soda bread; toast and toss with fresh fruit, herbs and leafy greens for a crunchy salad; sprinkle on soups, stews and casseroles.

SEE: FRUIT & NUT MUESLI, P42; BERRY & COCONUT PORRIDGE, P43; ON-THE-GO GRANOLA BARS, P40; BANANA, OAT & BLACKBERRY MUFFINS, P68; ROSEMARY OATCAKES, P63; WATERCRESS SOUP WITH CHEESY OATCAKES, P88.

Cinnamon

- ✔ Lowers blood sugar levels
- ✔ Supports liver function
- ✔ Boosts metabolism
- ✔ Lowers cholesterol
- ✔ Decreases memory loss and enhances brain activity
- ✔ Improves circulation
- ✔ Reduces joint pain
- ✔ Reduces the risk of tooth decay and gum disease
- ✔ Helps prevent bone loss
- ✔ Eases palpitations
- ✔ Raises libido
- ✔ Discourages cellulite

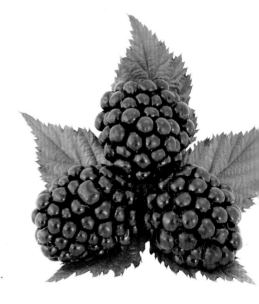

Just a little cinnamon, eaten daily, can play a strong role in preventing many of the problems that accompany ageing, including reducing inflammation that can affect the heart, skin, brain and joints. It helps to normalize blood sugar levels, which play a role in excess weight and diabetes, and also has a calming effect that can encourage restful sleep and even ease palpitations. Its antibacterial properties help to ensure good oral health.

It's rich in...

- → Polyphenols, antioxidants which promote heart health and lower the risk of cardiovascular disease, as well as reducing inflammation
- → MCHP (methylhydroxychalcone polymer) which enhances the effect of insulin, reduces blood sugar, lowers cholesterol and encourages a sense of calm
- → Sulphur which supports the liver to improve digestion and energy levels, while discouraging cellulite
- → Manganese to build bones, blood and other connective tissues; it also contains a chemical which stops bones from breaking down

- → Calcium to encourage restful sleep, support bone health and a healthy nervous system

Use in... porridge; stir into warm, freshly pressed apple juice; use to flavour unsweetened fruit purées and serve with live yogurt; add to tagines, chillies and stews to bring out the flavour; steep cinnamon sticks in boiling water to make a nutritious, stimulating tea; sprinkle over mashed bananas or puréed apples and pears and use as a spread; stir-fry with chickpeas.

SEE: BERRY & BRAZIL NUT SMOOTHIE, P39; ON-THE-GO GRANOLA BARS, P40; CARROT CRISPS WITH HONEY YOGURT DIP, P58; BANANA, OAT & BLACKBERRY MUFFINS, P68; CARROT & BEETROOT TABBOULEH, P78; CHICKEN MOLE, P92; GUAVA-GLAZED PORK TENDERLOIN, P96; BAKED HONEY, CARDAMOM & CINNAMON FIGS, P112; FRUIT SALSA & CINNAMON CRISPS, P114; CRANBERRY ICE CREAM WITH DARK CHOCOLATE, P118.

Blackberries

✔ Help digestion and ease constipation
✔ Balance blood sugar levels
✔ Relieve pain and protect eyesight
✔ Promote healthy liver function
✔ Improve mood, memory and libido
✔ Strengthen bones and teeth
✔ Protect against cardiovascular disease
✔ Discourage cellulite

Blackberries are full of age-defying anti-oxidants. They fight inflammation and the high fibre content promotes healthy digestion and lowers cholesterol and blood pressure.

They are rich in...

→ Folate to fight cardiovascular disease and memory loss; to produce serotonin for good mood and healthy sleep
→ Anthocyanins which ease inflammation and improve circulation, muscle tone and brain function
→ Fibre to balance blood sugar and help digestion and liver function, which will discourage cellulite
→ Vitamin K which is needed for the nervous system, brain function and strong bones and teeth
→ Vitamin C to prevent arthritis, macular degeneration and joint problems, and to produce collagen for better hair and skin

Use in... salads with walnuts, tart apples and feta cheese; bakes such as muffins, scones and fruit breads; fruit compotes and crumbles; smoothies with almond milk and honey; roast with pork or duck; braise with red cabbage or fennel.

SEE: BERRY & COCONUT PORRIDGE, P43; BANANA, OAT & BLACKBERRY MUFFINS, P68; BLACKBERRY BRÛLÉES, P123; APPLE & BLACKBERRY COMPOTE WITH ALMOND SCONES, P124; GUAVA ICE CREAM WITH BLACKBERRY COULIS, P120.

Broccoli

✔ Protects eyesight
✔ Reduces memory loss
✔ Supports bone health
✔ Boosts production of red blood cells
✔ Raises energy levels
✔ Supports liver function
✔ Protects against heart disease
✔ Reduces inflammation and cellulite
✔ Improves digestion

Rich in A, B-complex, C and K vitamins, iron, zinc, phosphorus, calcium, potassium and protein, broccoli has anti-inflammatory properties and fibre to stabilize blood sugar. It may even help reverse the effects of ageing.

It's rich in...

→ Sulforaphane which protects against cancer and free radical damage in hair, bones, skin, heart and joints, and improves blood pressure
→ Folate and calcium for bone health and restful sleep, and to combat cognitive decline
→ Lignans to fight cancers and heart disease, boost immunity and brain health
→ Carotenoids which support eye and heart health

Use in... stir-fries with spring onions and light soy sauce; lightly steamed or raw florets in salads; add to the final cooking stage of soups, stews and casseroles; frittatas and omelettes; raw with healthy dips such as guacamole and hummus; steam and purée with pine nuts, pecorino cheese, lemon juice and olive oil for pesto.

SEE: PESTO BROCCOLI WITH POACHED EGGS, P80; BROCCOLI & RED PEPPER FRITTATA, P46; TOASTED QUINOA, TUNA & LENTIL SALAD, P98; BROCCOLI SALAD WITH DILL & PINE NUTS, P76; BUTTERNUT, BROCCOLI & MUSHROOM GRATIN, P105.

Sardines

✔ Help prevent blindness
✔ Strengthen bones and ease joint pain
✔ Support cardiovascular health
✔ Improve memory and ward off some forms of dementia
✔ Reduce wrinkles and thinning of skin
✔ Lift mood

Sardines are a great source of omega-3 fatty acids which have lots of anti-ageing benefits, such as the health of the heart and brain. Their other nutrients include vitamin D, essential for strong bones and teeth.

They are rich in...

→ Vitamin B12 which is needed for healthy circulation, energy and heart health
→ Vitamin D for strong bones and teeth, and the prevention of osteoporosis; also aids the absorption of calcium
→ Phosphorus, a mineral which is required to strengthen the bone matrix
→ Vital omega-3 oils which maintain heart health, reduce mental decline, prevent degeneration of the eyes, reduce wrinkles by improving elasticity, ease inflammation and restore lustre to hair
→ Selenium, a known anti-ageing mineral which also helps to lift mood

Use in... salads with cucumber, Romaine lettuce and feta cheese; grill or barbecue sprinkled with fresh herbs, lemon and olive oil; mash into tomato pasta sauces; top with chopped fresh tomatoes, basil and toasted pine nuts; crush on wholegrain crackers or rye bread and sprinkle with lemon juice and black pepper; marinate in fresh herbs, garlic and saffron and grill.

SEE: ROASTED CHILLI & LEMON SARDINES, P84; AVOCADO & SARDINE SALAD WITH ZESTY DRESSING, P72.

Dark chocolate

✔ Lifts mood, energy and alertness
✔ Encourages relaxation
✔ Reduces pain
✔ Lowers blood pressure and cholesterol
✔ Balances blood sugar
✔ Reduces wrinkles and dry skin
✔ Prevents tooth decay
✔ Enhances brain and heart health
✔ Helps angina

The nutrients in dark chocolate work to slow the ageing process on all levels, lift mood, improve alertness and relaxation, and contain chemicals to fight tooth decay. Its resveratrol can increase the life span of cells by up to 80 per cent. Choose chocolate with at least 70 per cent cocoa solids.

It's rich in...

→ Theobromine which combats fatigue, boosts brain power, mildly stimulates the heart and lowers blood pressure
→ Procyanidins to relax blood vessels and aid circulation, heart health and virility
→ Polyphenols which lower cholesterol
→ Flavonoids which reduce inflammation of the skin caused by exposure to UV light, and also increase circulation to the skin, making it moister, more supple and less wrinkled
→ Copper to help hair keep its colour

Use in... spicy chillies and curries to deepen flavour; melted in smoothies with banana and live yogurt; grate over porridge, fresh fruit or yogurt; snack on a handful of chocolate-covered brazil nuts; eat a couple of small squares as an after-dinner treat.

SEE: CHICKEN MOLE, P92; BANANAS WITH SPICED CHOCOLATE, P116; CHOCOLATE PUDDLE PUDDINGS, P115; CRANBERRY ICE CREAM WITH DARK CHOCOLATE, P118.

Avocados

✔ Reduce inflammation and age spots
✔ Prevent wrinkles, dry skin and hair
✔ Boost collagen production
✔ Encourage heart and brain health
✔ Lower cholesterol and blood sugar
✔ Improve digestion
✔ Promote healthy sleep and relaxation

A source of good fats, avocados are packed with nutrients which can improve heart and brain health, and also ease pain, encourage relaxation, memory and healthy sleep, and prevent degeneration of hair, skin and joints.

They are rich in...

→ Oleic acid which increases good cholesterol and lowers bad cholesterol
→ Potassium which protects the heart, circulatory system and nervous system, reduces the risk of high blood pressure, angina and stroke, raises energy levels, improves mood, and decreases pain and inflammation
→ Omega-3 fatty acids for heart, brain and skin health
→ Magnesium to promote healthy sleep and relaxation and boost immunity
→ Vitamins A and C which slow down the effects of ageing, maintain eyesight and boost collagen formation in the skin

Use in... tricolore salads with tomato and mozzarella; mash on toast instead of butter, or in sandwiches instead of mayonnaise; guacamole with fresh crudités; warm and cold salads, or serve with a dressing on top; puréed in smoothies with vanilla, live yogurt and honey.

SEE: BAKED AVOCADO EGG CUPS, P44; AVOCADO
& TOMATO TOSTADOS, P60; CHILLED AVOCADO
SOUP, P90; AVOCADO & SARDINE SALAD WITH
ZESTY DRESSING, P72.

Guavas

✔ Balance weight
✔ Ease constipation and encourage healthy digestion
✔ Enhance brain function
✔ Improve skin quality and eyesight
✔ Lower blood pressure and cholesterol
✔ Prevent gum disease

This nutritious Asian fruit is bursting with protein to help repair and restore tissues in the body. With no cholesterol, few calories and little sugar, it's ideal for a healthy diet. Its astringent and antibacterial compounds help prevent gum disease and tooth decay.

They are rich in...

→ Antioxidants and phenols which protect against heart disease and stroke
→ Prebiotics and fibre to encourage healthy digestion
→ Potassium to ease palpitations and lower blood pressure
→ Vitamin C to improve immunity, heart health, eyes and skin
→ B vitamins for relaxation, increased energy and improved sleep
→ Vitamin A for eye health and reduced risk of cataracts and macular degeneration

Use in... smoothies with berries and bananas; stir into live yogurt and top with cinnamon and a swirl of maple syrup; use in juices with fresh vegetables and fruits; add to salads with feta, chicken and nuts; toss into curries and tagines; chop with mango in fresh salsas; or simply eat fresh and ripe as a snack.

SEE: GUAVA & GINGER SMOOTHIE, P38; GUAVA
& MANGO SHAKE, P57; GUAVA-GLAZED PORK
TENDERLOIN, P96; GUAVA ICE CREAM WITH
BLACKBERRY COULIS, P120.

Quinoa

✔ Lifts mood
✔ Aids restful sleep and reduces fatigue
✔ Balances blood sugar levels
✔ Eases chronic pain
✔ Protects hair and restores colour
✔ Reduces age spots and wrinkles
✔ Improves memory and cognition
✔ Encourages healthy digestion
✔ Supports bone health
✔ Reduces inflammation

Quinoa is a nutritious, protein-rich seed full of B vitamins, fibre and iron to lift energy levels and mood. It contains all of the amino acids needed to create and protect cells, and is rich in antioxidants and omega oils.

It's rich in...

→ Amino acids to nourish the hair follicles and promote growth; tyrosine can encourage re-pigmentation of the hair
→ Melatonin to encourage restful sleep and healthy sleep patterns
→ Lysine to help your body absorb calcium to protect bones; produces elastin and collagen for healthy skin
→ Fibre to balance blood sugar levels, support the liver and healthy digestion, ease constipation and stabilize mood

Use in... soups, casseroles, stir-fries and stews; instead of rice or couscous in salads; as a bed for curries, tagines, chillies and roasted vegetable dishes; salad with dried cherries, pistachios, artichoke hearts, lemon juice, olive oil and parsley; loaves and cakes with dried fruit and nuts; breakfast cereal with almond or soya milk and fresh fruit.

SEE: POACHED EGGS ON QUINOA HASH BROWNS, P49; MEDITERRANEAN STUFFED PEPPERS, P82; ASPARAGUS & PEA QUINOA RISOTTO, P99; TOASTED QUINOA, TUNA & LENTIL SALAD, P98.

Garlic

✔ Helps immunity and digestion
✔ Lifts mood and energy levels
✔ Supports the nervous system
✔ Essential for heart and brain health
✔ Necessary for skin and eye health
✔ Regulates blood sugar levels
✔ Encourages restful sleep and oral health
✔ Reduces blood pressure and cholesterol

Garlic can prevent cardiovascular disease, arthritis and cataracts, improve circulation, rejuvenate skin and increase energy levels. Studies also suggest that it prevents and delays chronic diseases that occur with age.

It's rich in...

→ Vitamin B6 which encourages healthy iron levels to boost energy and mood and keep the heart and brain functioning optimally; prevents premature grey hair
→ Sulphur to produce collagen, which fights wrinkles and inflammation, protects from free radicals and maintains healthy gums
→ Allicin to promote circulation, which aids skin, heart, memory and hair growth, and reduces blood pressure and inflammation
→ Selenium and vitamin C which can help to delay and reverse the signs of ageing

Use in... salad dressings, stews, dips, soups and casseroles; roast and spread on whole grain bread or oatcakes; curries; pasta sauces; aioli; flavour steamed vegetables; spread on fish; bake with shallots in sherry; rub into the skin of a whole chicken and fill the cavity with garlic cloves; creamy yogurt sauces served with leafy greens, lamb or poultry.

SEE: VIRTUALLY EVERY SAVOURY DIP OR COOKED RECIPE IN THIS BOOK, ESPECIALLY CARAMELIZED GARLIC TART, P106; AIOLI WITH CRISPBREADS & CRUDITES, P54; SPAGHETTI WITH OLIVE OIL, GARLIC & CHILLI, P111.

Eggs

- ✔ Regulate mood
- ✔ Encourage concentration and alertness
- ✔ Stabilize blood sugar
- ✔ Promote sleep and relaxation
- ✔ Maintain healthy skin and hair
- ✔ Protect eyesight
- ✔ Support brain and heart health
- ✔ Help prevent bone loss
- ✔ Boost metabolism

One of the most important sources of high-quality protein, eggs contain amino acids that are essential for the building and repair of body tissues, such as skin and muscles. They provide a great source of sustainable energy which will help to balance weight and beat fatigue. What's more, they are fabulous for heart health and help to reverse the symptoms of stress, including easing palpitations.

They are rich in...
- → Betaine and choline which are essential for healthy functioning of the brain, nervous system and cardiovascular system
- → Vitamin D to encourage healthy bones and teeth
- → Lutein and zeaxanthin which are required for healthy eyesight

Use in... omelettes with spinach, herbs and mushrooms; simply boil for an easy, nutritious snack; scramble with chives and top with smoked salmon or other oily fish; chop and add to salads; poach and serve with spinach, asparagus or grilled portabello mushrooms; use in frittatas with feta and peas, courgettes and other green vegetables.

SEE: HUEVOS RANCHEROS, P48; BAKED AVOCADO EGG CUPS, P44; POACHED EGGS ON QUINOA HASH BROWNS, P49; BROCCOLI & RED PEPPER FRITTATA, P46; BANANA, OAT & BLACKBERRY MUFFINS, P68; AOILI WITH CRISPBREADS & CRUDITÉS, P54; PESTO BROCCOLI WITH POACHED EGGS, P80; FENNEL & MUSHROOM TARTS, P86; CARAMELIZED GARLIC TART, P106; BLACKBERRY BRÛLÉES, P123.

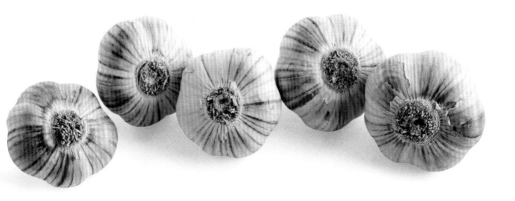

WHAT'S YOUR PROBLEM?

These functional foods contain the nutrients that target specific problems related to the effects of ageing, both internal and external. Decide which symptoms affect you and choose from the foods and recipes that can relieve them. These icons are used throughout the recipe section to highlight which recipes can help combat which symptoms.

Wrinkles

Cranberries, guavas, sardines, tomatoes, avocados, broccoli, pomegranates, dark chocolate, carrots, leafy greens, fennel, aubergines, brazil nuts, red peppers, eggs, quinoa, olive oil, garlic, cinnamon, blackberries, oats, watercress, tuna
Recipes include:
Rosemary oatcakes, p63; Banana, oat & blackberry muffins, p68; Toasted quinoa, tuna & lentil salad, p98; Guava ice cream with blackberry coulis, p120.

Age spots

Cranberries, olive oil, sardines, dark chocolate, broccoli, avocados, brazil nuts, red peppers, guavas, aubergines, pomegranates, carrots, quinoa, cinnamon, tuna, watercress, fennel
Recipes include:
Spicy brazil nuts, p56; Fennel & mushroom tarts, p86; Chicken mole, p92; Guava-glazed pork tenderloin, p96.

Dry skin

Sardines, avocados, dark chocolate, red peppers, carrots, pomegranates, eggs, quinoa, olive oil, cranberries, blackberries, leafy greens, aubergines, broccoli, brazil nuts, guavas, fennel, garlic
Recipes include:
Baked avocado egg cups, p44; Roasted chilli & lemon sardines, p84; Broccoli salad with dill & pine nuts, p76; Tuna with peppers & fennel gratin, p104.

Tooth decay

Cranberries, dark chocolate, guavas, cinnamon, garlic, watercress, tuna, olive oil, eggs, sardines, broccoli
Recipes include:
On-the-go granola bars, p40; Watercress soup with cheesy oatcakes, p88; Sesame-crusted tuna with ginger dressing, p102; Cranberry ice cream with dark chocolate, p118.

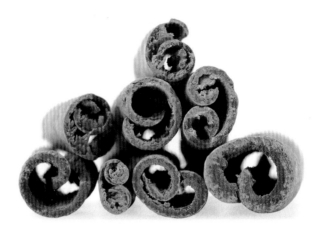

Spider veins

Sardines, tomatoes, pomegranate, dark chocolate, tuna, avocados, oats, aubergines, red peppers, eggs, carrots, quinoa, cinnamon, olive oil, garlic, blackberries, broccoli, leafy greens, brazil nuts, fennel, guavas, watercress
Recipes include:
Guava & ginger smoothie, p38; Citrus olives, p50; Aubergine, chickpea & paneer curry, p110; Pomegranate panna cotta, p122.

Lack of libido

Dark chocolate, carrots, oats, watercress, brazil nuts, blackberries, cinnamon, garlic
Recipes include:
Berry & coconut porridge, p43; Carrot & beetroot tabbouleh, p78; Spicy brazil nuts, p56; Caramelized garlic tart, p106.

Thinning hair

Sardines, avocados, aubergines, red peppers, carrots, pomegranates, eggs, brazil nuts, olive oil, fennel, oats, blackberries, watercress, tuna, broccoli, quinoa, tomatoes, garlic
Recipes include:
Smoky aubergine dip, p53; Carrot, coriander & lentil soup, p91; Fennel-roasted lamb with figs, p94; Hearty ratatouille, p108.

Grey hair

Quinoa, carrots, dark chocolate, tomatoes, eggs, broccoli, garlic, red peppers, brazil nuts, blackberries, tuna, watercress, sardines
Recipes include:
Broccoli & red pepper frittata, p46; Asparagus & pea quinoa risotto, p99; Butternut, broccoli & mushroom gratin, p105; Apple & blackberry compote with almond scones, p124.

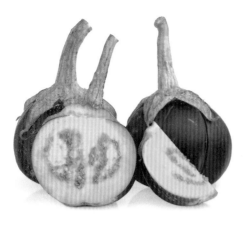
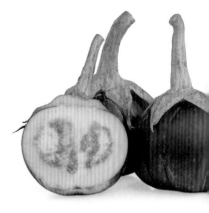

Weak bones

Sardines, broccoli, pomegranates, eggs, blackberries, quinoa, watercress, olive oil, cinnamon, tomatoes, tuna, aubergines
Recipes include:
Poached eggs on quinoa hash browns, p49; Bruschetta with tomatoes & basil, p62; Roasted chilli & lemon sardines, p84; Guava-glazed pork tenderloin, p96.

Poor circulation

Cranberries, sardines, dark chocolate, carrots, aubergines, red peppers, cinnamon, pomegranates, eggs, blackberries, garlic, broccoli
Recipes include:
Blueberry pomegranate smoothie, p36; Spiced raisin & cranberry cookies, p64; Aubergine & sesame noodle salad, p70; Blackberry brûlées, p123.

Eyesight

Sardines, avocado, aubergines, red peppers, tomatoes, pomegranate, eggs, carrots, guava, fennel, blackberries, tuna, broccoli
Recipes Include:
Baked avocado egg cups, p44; Carrot & Puy lentil salad, p75; Avocado & sardine salad with zesty dressing, p72; Guava ice cream with blackberry coulis, p120.

Poor sleep

Dark chocolate, avocados, red peppers, eggs, guavas, oats, blackberries, tuna, quinoa, broccoli, cinnamon, garlic
Recipes include:
Huevos rancheros, p48; Chilled avocado soup, p90; Butternut, broccoli & mushroom gratin, p105; Bananas with spiced chocolate, p116.

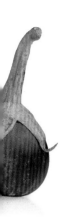

Low energy

Sardines, guavas, dark chocolate, avocados, oats, aubergines, red peppers, garlic, pomegranates, eggs, brazil nuts, carrots, fennel, watercress, tuna, broccoli, quinoa

Recipes include:
Fruit & nut muesli, p42; Aioli with crispbreads & crudités, p54; Fennel & cumin Waldorf salad, p74; Tuna with peppers & fennel gratin, p104.

Joint pain & stiffness

Dark chocolate, cranberries, oats, sardines, avocados, red peppers, tuna, pomegranates, eggs, brazil nuts, olive oil, cinnamon, tomatoes, blackberries

Recipes include:
Avocado & tomato tostados, p60; Avocado & sardine salad with zesty dressing, p72; Chicken mole, p92; Pomegranate panna cotta, p122.

Poor memory & forgetfulness

Cranberries, olive oil, sardines, dark chocolate, quinoa aubergines, red peppers, avocado, pomegranate, eggs, brazil nuts, oats, blackberries, watercress, tuna, broccoli, cinnamon

Recipes Include:
Berry & brazil nut smoothie, p39; Cranberry muffins, p69; Toasted quinoa, tuna & lentil salad, p98; Chocolate puddle puddings, p115.

Cellulite

Cranberries, dark chocolate, red peppers, tomatoes, aubergines, fennel, pomegranates, eggs, carrots, guavas, cinnamon, blackberries, garlic, broccoli, quinoa

Recipes include:
Carrot crisps with honey yogurt dip, p58; Pesto broccoli with poached eggs, p80; Mediterranean stuffed peppers, p82; Baked honey, cardamom & cinnamon figs, p112.

PUTTING IT ALL TOGETHER

Meal Planner	Monday	Tuesday	Wednesday
Breakfast	Fruit & nut muesli, p42	On-the-go granola bars, p40	Berry & coconut porridge, p43
Morning snack	Guava & mango shake, p57	Spicy brazil nuts, p56	Bruschetta with tomatoes & basil, p62
Lunch	Carrot & Puy lentil salad, p75	Aubergine & sesame noodle salad, p70	Pesto broccoli with poached eggs, p80
Afternoon snack	Carrot crisps with honey yogurt dip, p58	Aioli with crispbreads & crudités, p54	Citrus olives, p50
Dinner	Spaghetti with olive oil, garlic & chilli, p111	Tuna with peppers & fennel gratin, p104	Miso aubergines with rice noodles, p100
Dessert	Blackberry brûlées, p123	Cranberry ice cream with dark chocolate, p118	Baked honey, cardamom & cinnamon figs, p112

WEEK 1

Thursday	**Friday**	**Saturday**	**Sunday**
Baked avocado egg cups, p44	Guava & ginger smoothie, p38	Huevos rancheros, p48	Poached eggs on quinoa hash browns, p49
Smoky aubergine dip, p53	Spiced raisin & cranberry cookies, p64	Carrot & lentil muffins, p66	Fresh pomegranate
Gazpacho, p83	Broccoli salad with dill & pine nuts, p76	Mediterranean stuffed peppers, p82	Watercress soup with cheesy oatcakes, p88
Cranberry muffins, p69	Avocado & tomato tostados, p60	Greek feta & mint dip, p52	Citrus olives, p50
Toasted quinoa, tuna & lentil salad, p98	Caramelized garlic tart, p106	Guava-glazed pork tenderloin, p96	Chicken mole, p92
Pomegranate panna cotta, p122	Bananas with spiced chocolate, p116	Fruit salsa & cinnamon crisps, p114	Apple & blackberry compote with almond scones, p124

Meal Planner	Monday	Tuesday	Wednesday
Breakfast	Berry & coconut porridge, p43	Berry & brazil nut smoothie, p39	On-the-go granola bars, p40
Morning snack	Spicy brazil nuts, p56	Spiced raisin & cranberry cookies, p64	A few brazil nuts covered in dark chocolate
Lunch	Avocado & sardine salad with zesty dressing, p72	Fennel & mushroom tarts, p86	Chilled avocado soup, p90
Afternoon snack	Bruschetta with tomatoes & basil, p62	Carrot crisps with honey yogurt dip, p58	Aioli with crispbreads & crudités, p54
Dinner	Asparagus & pea quinoa risotto, p99	Sesame-crusted tuna with ginger dressing, p102	Hearty ratatouille, p108
Dessert	Guava ice cream with blackberry coulis, p120	Chocolate puddle puddings, p115	Pomegranate panna cotta, p122

WEEK 2

	Thursday	Friday	Saturday	Sunday
	Fruit & nut muesli, p42	Blueberry pomegranate smoothie, p36	Broccoli & red pepper frittata, p46	Baked avocado egg cups, p44
	Smoky aubergine dip, p53	Avocado & tomato tostados, p60	Carrot & lentil muffins, p66	Spicy brazil nuts, p56
	Fennel & cumin Waldorf salad, p74	Carrot, coriander & lentil soup, p91	Roasted chilli & lemon sardines, p84	Carrot & beetroot tabbouleh, p78
	Carrot & lentil muffins, p66	Rosemary oatcakes, p63	Greek feta & mint dip, p52	Spiced raisin & cranberry cookies, p64
	Butternut, broccoli & mushroom gratin, p105	Aubergine, chickpea & paneer curry, p110	Fennel-roasted lamb with figs, p94	Toasted quinoa, tuna & lentil salad, p98
	Baked honey, cardamom & cinnamon figs, p112	Fruit salsa & cinnamon crisps, p114	Pomegranate panna cotta, p122	Cranberry ice cream with dark chocolate, p118

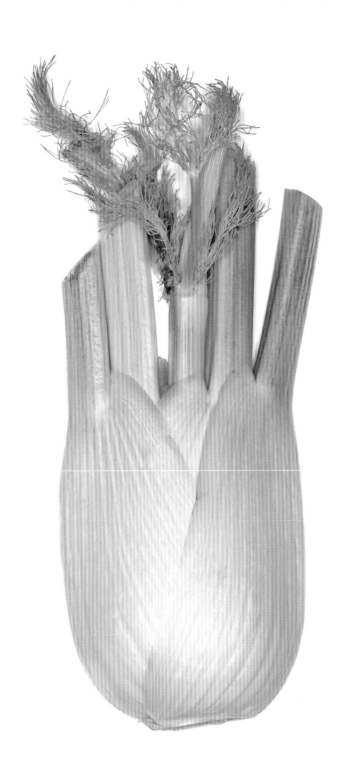

YOUNG
RECIPES

BLUEBERRY POMEGRANATE SMOOTHIE

This fresh, fruity smoothie has superior antioxidant levels and is guaranteed to lift your mood and energy levels.

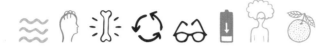

Preparation time: 5 minutes
Serves 4
....

400 g (13 oz) **blueberries**
600 ml (1 pint) **pomegranate juice**
50 g (2 oz) **pomegranate seeds**
100 g (3½ oz) **baby spinach**
2 **bananas**, peeled and cut into chunks
10 **ice cubes**

Place all the ingredients in a blender or food processor and blitz until smooth. Serve icy cold.
....

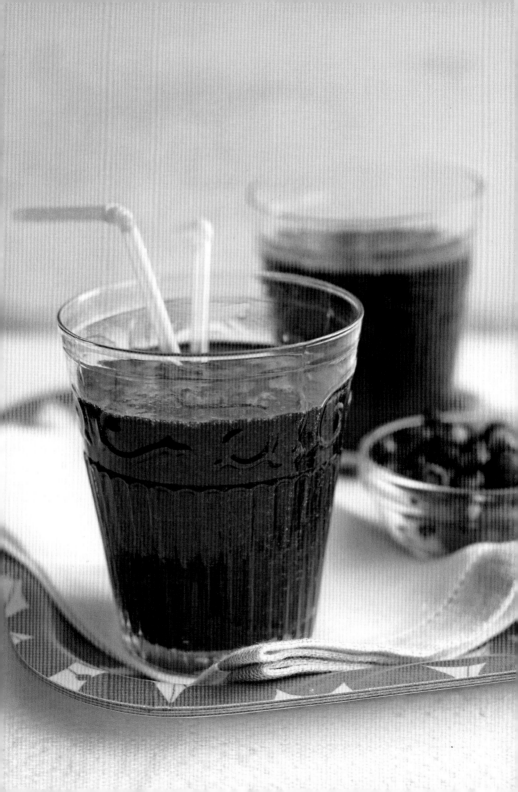

GUAVA & GINGER SMOOTHIE

Kick-start the day with circulation-boosting ginger and a wealth of antioxidants to protect your cells against the ravages of time.

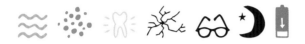

Preparation time: 10 minutes
Serves 4
....

2 **guavas**, peeled, deseeded
and cut into chunks
½ **pineapple**, peeled, cored
and cut into chunks
2 **bananas**, peeled and cut into chunks
2 cm (¾ inch) piece of fresh **root ginger**,
peeled and sliced
400 ml (13 fl oz) **almond milk**
10 **ice cubes**

Place all the ingredients in a blender or food processor and blitz until smooth and creamy. Serve icy cold.

....

BERRY & BRAZIL NUT SMOOTHIE

Rich in healthy proteins, omega oils and antioxidants, this fresh, filling smoothie is a pick-me-up that will keep you up!

Preparation time: 10 minutes
Serves 4
....

200 g (7 oz) fresh or frozen **strawberries**, hulled
200 g (7 oz) fresh or frozen **raspberries**
200 g (7 oz) fresh or frozen **blackberries**
100 g (3½ oz) raw **brazil nuts**
1 **banana**, peeled and cut into chunks
1 tsp **ground cinnamon**
300 ml (½ pint) **soya milk**
1 tbsp **honey**
10 **ice cubes**

Place all the ingredients in a blender or food processor and blitz for about 5 minutes until smooth. Serve icy cold.

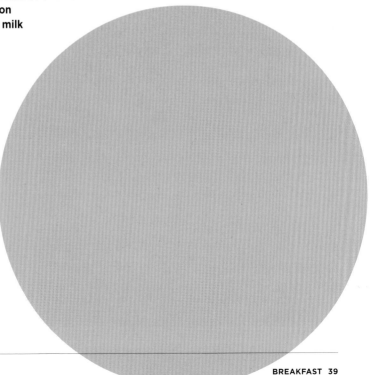

ON-THE-GO GRANOLA BARS

There's no need to make compromises when eating breakfast on the run: these granola bars pack a punch with cinnamon, oats, fruit, nuts and seeds.

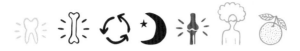

Preparation time: 5 minutes
Cooking time: 20 minutes
Makes 9

75 g (3 oz) **butter**, plus extra for greasing
75 ml (3 fl oz) clear **honey**
½ tsp **ground cinnamon**
100 g (3½ oz) **soft dried apricots**, roughly chopped
50 g (2 oz) **soft dried papaya** or **mango**, roughly chopped
50 g (2 oz) **raisins**
4 tbsps **mixed seeds** (pumpkin, sesame and sunflower)
50 g (2 oz) **pecan nuts**, roughly broken
150 g (5 oz) **porridge oats**

Place the butter and honey in a saucepan and bring to the boil, stirring continuously, until the mixture bubbles.

Add the cinnamon, dried fruit, seeds and pecan nuts, then stir and heat for 1 minute. Remove from the heat and add the porridge oats. Stir well, then transfer the mixture to a greased shallow 20 cm (8 inch) square baking tin and press down well.

Place in a preheated oven, 190°C (375°F), Gas Mark 5, for 15 minutes until the top is just beginning to brown. Leave to cool in the tin, then cut into 9 granola squares or bars. Store in an airtight container for up to a week.

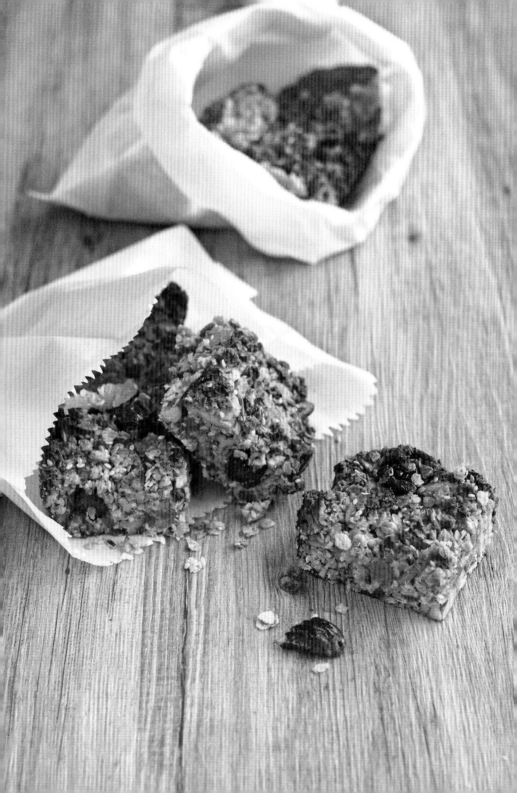

FRUIT & NUT MUESLI

The brazil nuts in this muesli provide age-defying selenium, the seeds provide omega-3s and the cranberries help maintain your teeth and skin. Divine!

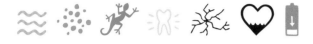

Preparation time: 5 minutes
Serves 4
....

200 g (7 oz) **porridge oats**
50 g (2 oz) **dried cranberries**
50 g (2 oz) **soft dried apricots**, chopped
50 g (2 oz) **dates**, chopped
50 g (2 oz) **pecan nuts**, chopped
50 g (2 oz) **brazil nuts**, chopped
3–4 tbsps **mixed seeds** (sunflower, pumpkin and flax seeds)

To serve
milk
live natural yogurt
chopped fresh **fruit**

Mix together all the dry ingredients. Divide between 4 serving bowls and serve with milk, yogurt and fresh fruit.
....

BERRY & COCONUT PORRIDGE

Bursting with B vitamins, insoluble fibre and antioxidants, this is the most delicious porridge you'll ever taste.

Preparation time: 5 minutes
Cooking time: 10 minutes
Serves 4
....

200 g (7 oz) **porridge oats**
3 tbsps **unsweetened desiccated coconut**, plus extra to scatter
600 ml (1 pint) **milk** or **soya milk**
600 ml (1 pint) **water**
4 tbsps **live natural yogurt**
200 g (7 oz) **berries** (blackberries, blueberries, raspberries and strawberries)
4 tbsps clear **honey**

Place the oats and coconut in a saucepan with the milk and measurement water. Bring to the boil, then reduce the heat and simmer for about 8 minutes until thick and creamy, stirring often.
....

Pour into 4 bowls and stir a swirl of the yogurt into each. Top with the berries and a drizzle of honey, then scatter with a little extra coconut.
....

BAKED AVOCADO EGG CUPS

Fresh coriander, crispy bacon, salsa, cheese or soured cream also make great toppings for this rejuvenating breakfast.

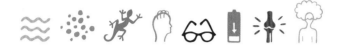

Preparation time: 5 minutes
Cooking time: 15 minutes
Serves 4
....

2 **avocados**, halved and pitted
4 **eggs**
½ tsp **cayenne pepper**
sea salt and **black pepper**
1 tbsp chopped **chives**, to garnish

Arrange the avocado halves, cut-sides up, in the holes of a muffin tin or in individual ramekins. Break an egg into each one, sprinkle with the cayenne pepper and season to taste.
....

Place in a preheated oven, 180°C (350°F), Gas Mark 4, for about 15 minutes or until the egg yolks are just set. Garnish with the chives and serve hot.
....

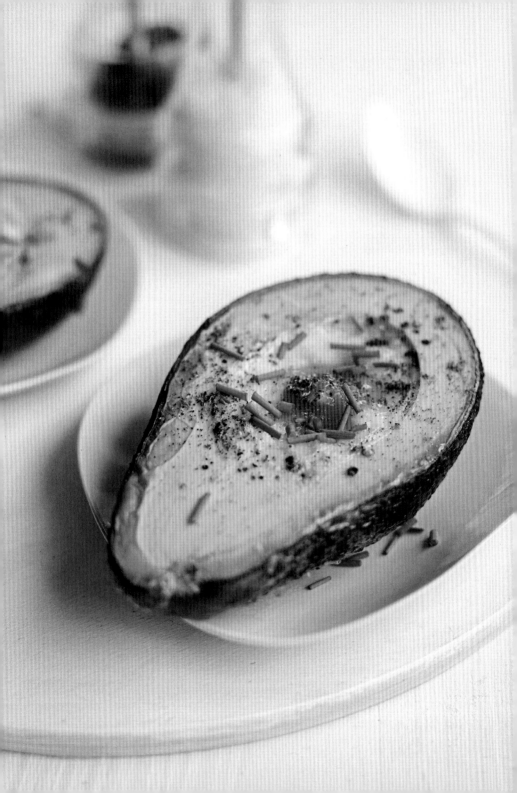

BROCCOLI & RED PEPPER FRITTATA

This tasty frittata makes a wonderful, nutritious breakfast for a lazy morning but could also be enjoyed warm or cold with salad for a light lunch.

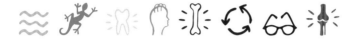

Preparation time: 10 minutes
Cooking time: 15 minutes
Serves 4

6 **eggs**
2 tbsps **milk**
100 g (3½ oz) strong **Cheddar cheese**, grated
1 head of **broccoli**, cut into florets
1 tbsp **olive oil**
1 **red pepper**, cored, deseeded and thinly sliced
1 **leek**, white part only, thinly sliced
100 g (3½ oz) **cherry tomatoes**, quartered
sea salt and **black pepper**

Place the eggs and milk in a mixing bowl and beat until fluffy. Season to taste, add half the grated cheese and mix well. Set to one side.

Cook the broccoli florets in a saucepan of lightly salted boiling water for 1 minute, then refresh in cold water and drain well.

Heat the olive oil in a large, nonstick, ovenproof frying pan over a medium heat and add the red pepper and leek. Cook for about 2 minutes until the leek starts to soften, then add the broccoli and cherry tomatoes.

Cook for a further 2–3 minutes, season to taste then arrange the vegetables evenly over the base of the pan. Pour in the egg mixture and continue cooking for about 3 minutes until the egg sets around the edges.

Place the pan under a preheated medium-hot grill for 5 minutes until the frittata is golden and set. Sprinkle over the remaining cheese and return to the grill until it bubbles. Transfer the frittata to a plate and serve in wedges.

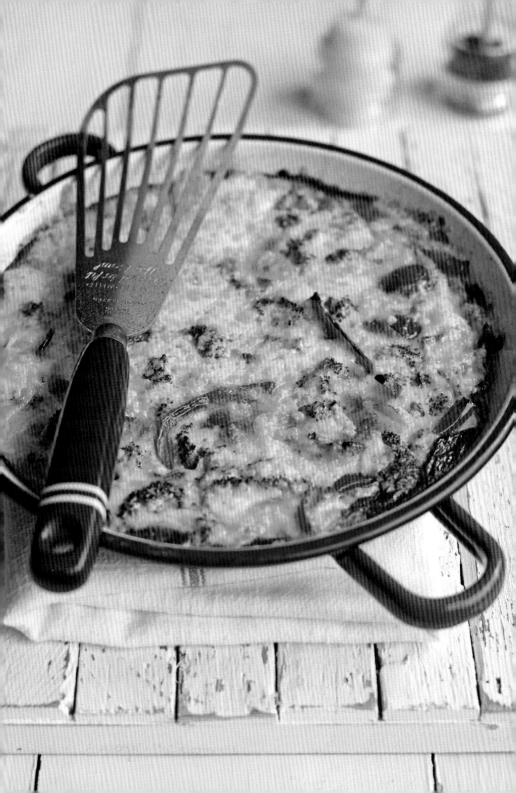

HUEVOS RANCHEROS

Full of rejuvenating garlic, red peppers and tomatoes, this Mexican classic is the perfect dish for a weekend breakfast all the family will want to share.

Preparation time: 10 minutes
Cooking time: 10 minutes
Serves 4
....

2 tbsps **olive oil**
1 large **onion**, diced
2 **red peppers**, cored, deseeded and diced
2 **garlic cloves**, crushed
¾ tsp **dried oregano**
400 g (13 oz) can **chopped tomatoes**
4 **eggs**
20 g (¾ oz) **feta cheese**, crumbled
sea salt and **black pepper**
seeded wholegrain bread, to serve

Heat the oil in a frying pan over a medium heat, add the onion, peppers, garlic and oregano and cook for 5 minutes.
....

Add the tomatoes, season to taste and |cook for a further 5 minutes. Pour the tomato mixture into a shallow ovenproof dish and make 4 dips in the mixture.
....

Crack the eggs into the dips, sprinkle with the feta and cook under a preheated hot grill for 3–4 minutes until the egg whites are set. Serve with chunks of seeded wholegrain bread to mop up the juices.
....

POACHED EGGS ON QUINOA HASH BROWNS

Full of protein and omega-3s, this tasty breakfast is packed with nutrients to keep you looking and feeling young.

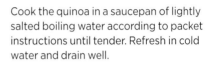

Preparation time: 15 minutes, plus chilling
Cooking time: 30 minutes
Serves 4

4 large **eggs**
1 tsp **vinegar**
sea salt and **black pepper**
2 **spring onions**, finely chopped, to garnish

Hash browns
100 g (3½ oz) **quinoa**
6 large **potatoes**, peeled and grated
1 **egg**, lightly beaten
1 tsp **ground cumin**
2 tbsps **olive oil**

Cook the quinoa in a saucepan of lightly salted boiling water according to packet instructions until tender. Refresh in cold water and drain well.

Place the grated potato on a clean tea towel, wrap tightly and using your hands squeeze out the excess moisture. Then transfer into a mixing bowl and add the egg, quinoa and cumin. Season to taste and mix together until well combined. Shape the mixture into 8 patties, arrange on a plate and chill in the refrigerator for 15 minutes or overnight.

Heat the olive oil in a large frying pan over a medium heat. Fry the patties in 2 batches for about 8 minutes each side until crisp, golden and cooked through. Drain on some kitchen paper.

Meanwhile, bring a saucepan of water to the boil and add the vinegar. Reduce the heat to a very low simmer and gently break the eggs into the water. Cook for about 5 minutes or until the whites are cooked through and the yolks are still runny.

Divide the hash browns between 4 plates and top with the eggs. Season to taste and sprinkle with the chopped spring onions before serving.

CITRUS OLIVES

A sunny snack with all the heart-healthy goodness of olive oil and the zing of fennel seeds, with a citrus twist.

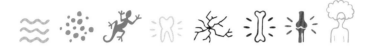

Preparation time: 5 minutes, plus marinating (optional)
Cooking time: 1 minutes
Serves 6
....

2 tsps **fennel seeds**
finely grated rind and juice of ½ **lemon**
finely grated rind and juice of ¼ **orange**
75 ml (3 fl oz) **olive oil**
400 g (13 oz) mixed **olives**

Place the fennel seeds in a small, dry frying pan over a medium heat and toast for about 30 seconds until they start to pop and emit an aroma. Remove from the frying pan and roughly crush.
....

Place the crushed fennel seeds, lemon and orange rind and juice and oil in a non-metallic bowl, then stir in the olives. Serve immediately or cover and leave to marinate overnight in a cool place before serving.
....

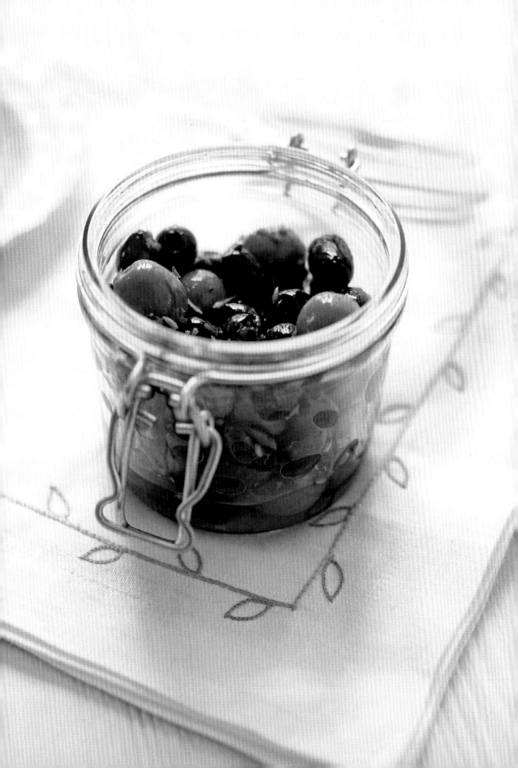

GREEK FETA & MINT DIP

A light and unbelievably tasty dip; this can also be served with wholewheat pittas, carrot sticks or broccoli florets.

Preparation time: 5 minutes
Serves 4
················

150 g (5 oz) **feta cheese**, crumbled
½ small **red onion**, finely chopped
handful of **mint** leaves, finely chopped
200 ml (7 fl oz) **live Greek yogurt**
black pepper
sliced **black olives**, to garnish

To serve
oatcakes
strips of **red pepper**

Mix the cheese with the onion, mint and yogurt, season with black pepper and stir gently to combine. Transfer to a bowl and scatter with a few sliced olives. Serve with oatcakes and strips of red pepper for dipping.

················

SMOKY AUBERGINE DIP

This delicious dip is rich in energy-boosting nutrients and will keep your skin and hair looking great.

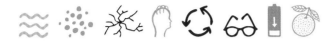

Preparation time: 20 minutes
Cooking time: 20 minutes
Serves 4-6
....

2 large **aubergines**
125 ml (4 fl oz) **live natural yogurt**
1 **garlic clove**, chopped
1 small **red chilli**, deseeded
and finely chopped
1 tsp **ground coriander**
½ tsp **ground cumin**
sea salt and **black pepper**
olive oil, to garnish
crudités or **wholemeal pitta breads**,
to serve

Place the whole aubergines on a baking sheet, prick all over with a fork and cook in a preheated oven, 230°C (450°F), Gas Mark 8, for 20 minutes or until the skins begin to blacken and the aubergines are soft right through.
....

Cut the aubergines in half and scrape all the soft flesh into the bowl of a food processor. Add the live yogurt, garlic, chilli, coriander and cumin. Blitz together until smooth and well combined, then season to taste. Transfer to a bowl and swirl a little olive oil over the top before serving with crudités or pittas.
....

AIOLI WITH CRISPBREADS & CRUDITÉS

This intensely garlicky dip is great for the circulation, heart, skin, memory, bones and hair. It will boost your energy levels and eradicate cellulite.

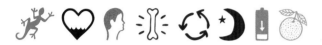

Preparation time: 10 minutes
Serves 4
....

3 **egg yolks**
5 **garlic cloves**, peeled
and roughly chopped
finely grated rind and juice of 1 **lemon**
1 tsp **mustard powder**
150 ml (5 fl oz) **olive oil**
sea salt and **black pepper**

To serve
crispbreads
crudités

Place the eggs yolks, garlic cloves, lemon rind and juice and mustard powder in the bowl of a food processer, season to taste and blitz until smooth and frothy.
....

With the motor still running, add the olive oil in a very slow but steady stream until the mixture becomes thick and unguent. Spoon into a bowl and serve with crispbreads and crudités for dipping.
....

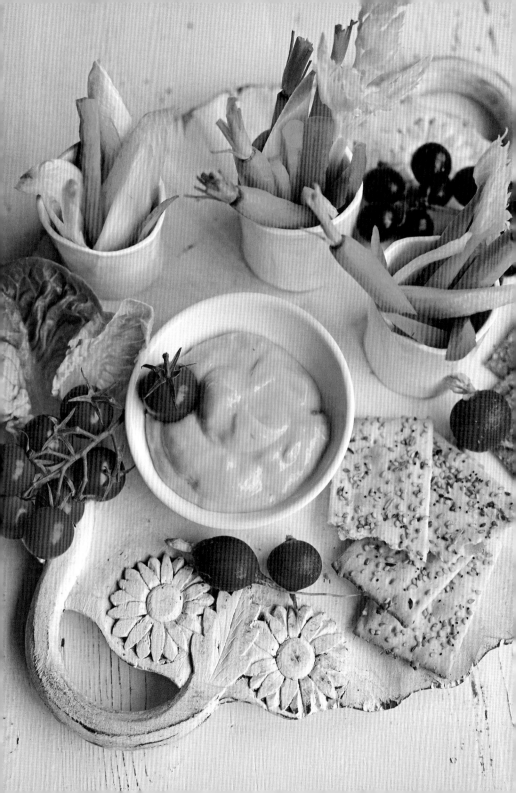

SPICY BRAZIL NUTS

Just a handful of these delicious nuts will boost energy levels and provide valuable omega oils to keep your skin and hair looking their best.

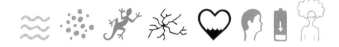

Preparation time: 5 minutes
Cooking time: 10 minutes
Serves 4-6
....

300 g (10 oz) raw **brazil nuts**
1 tbsp **rosemary** leaves, finely chopped
1 tsp **dark brown sugar**
1 tsp **sea salt**
1 tsp freshly ground **black pepper**
½ tsp **cayenne pepper**
2 tbsps **olive oil**

Arrange the brazil nuts on a baking sheet and place in a preheated oven, 180°C (350°F), Gas Mark 4, for 10 minutes or until they are lightly browned and fragrant.
....

Meanwhile, place the rosemary, sugar, salt, pepper, cayenne pepper and olive oil in a large bowl and mix well.
....

Tip the hot nuts into the flavoured oil, stir to coat and serve warm or cold. Store any leftover nuts in an airtight container for up to a week.
....

GUAVA & MANGO SHAKE

Bursting with fibre, antioxidants and protein, this will steady blood sugar levels and rejuvenate mind and body.

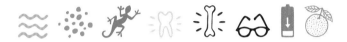

Preparation time: 10 minutes
Serves 4
....

2 **guavas**, peeled, deseeded
and cut into chunks
2 **mangos**, peeled, pitted
and cut into chunks
2 tbsps **coconut cream**
finely grated rind and juice of 1 **lemon**
2 tbsps **honey**
600 ml (1 pint) **skimmed milk** or **soya milk**
10 **ice cubes**

Place all the ingredients in a blender or food processor and blitz until smooth. Serve icy cold.
....

CARROT CRISPS WITH HONEY YOGURT DIP

These cinnamon carrot crisps are bursting with antioxidants and vitamin A to improve overall health, appearance and wellbeing.

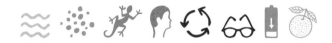

Preparation time: 10 minutes, plus cooling
Cooking time: 10 minutes
Serves 4

4 large **carrots**
1 tsp **ground cinnamon**
½ tsp **ground ginger**
½ tsp grated **nutmeg**
pinch of **sea salt**
pinch of **black pepper**
1 tbsp **olive oil**, plus extra to serve
150 ml (5 fl oz) **live Greek yogurt**
1 tbsp **honey**

Scrub the carrots then cut them into long thin strips using a vegetable peeler or a sharp knife. The thickness doesn't matter, as long as they are all similar.

Mix the cinnamon, ginger, nutmeg, salt, pepper and olive oil in a large mixing bowl. Add the carrot strips to the bowl and toss with your hands to coat evenly. Spread the strips out in a single layer on several baking sheets and place in a preheated oven, 220°C (428°F), Gas Mark 4, for about 10 minutes or until beginning to crisp. Set aside to cool.

Meanwhile, mix the yogurt and honey in a small bowl and drizzle over a swirl of olive oil. Serve with the crispy carrots.

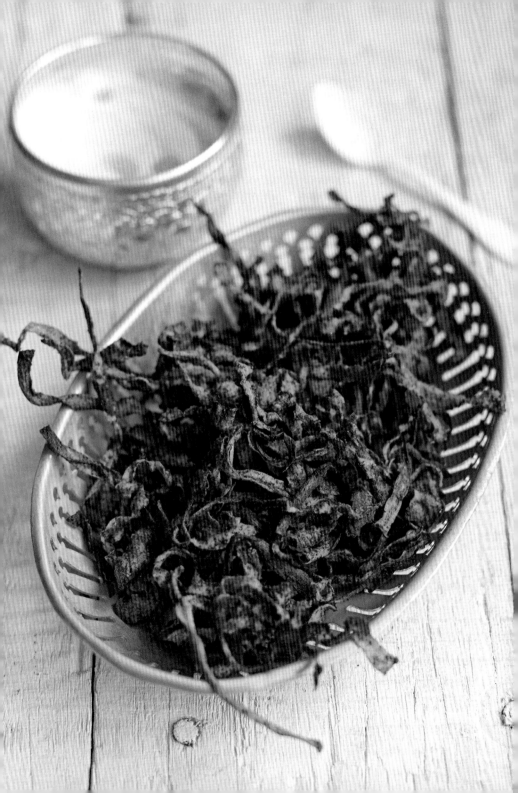

AVOCADO & TOMATO TOSTADOS

With lycopene, powerful antioxidants and omega-3s, this snack is perfect for beating wrinkles and grey hair.

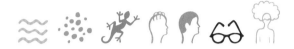

Preparation time: 15 minutes
Cooking time: 2 minutes
Serves 4
....

4 soft **corn tortillas**
1 tbsp **vegetable oil**
2 **avocados**, peeled and pitted
50 ml (2 fl oz) **live Greek yogurt**
2–3 tbsps **lime juice**
4 **tomatoes**, chopped
1 tbsp finely chopped **red onion**
1 tbsp **extra virgin olive oil**
handful of fresh **coriander**,
chopped, plus extra to garnish
sea salt and **black pepper**

Use a 5 cm (2 inch) biscuit cutter to stamp out rounds from the tortillas; alternatively, cut them into wedges. Brush them with the vegetable oil, place on a baking sheet under a preheated hot grill and cook for 1 minute on each side until crisp. Leave to cool.
....

Meanwhile, place the avocado flesh and live Greek yogurt in a food processor and blitz until smooth. Stir in 1 tablespoon of the lime juice and season to taste.
....

Place the tomatoes in a bowl with the onion and olive oil, add lime juice to taste, season and stir in the coriander.
....

Spoon a little of the avocado mixture on to each crispy tortilla, scatter over the tomato salsa and top with a little more coriander to garnish. Serve immediately.
....

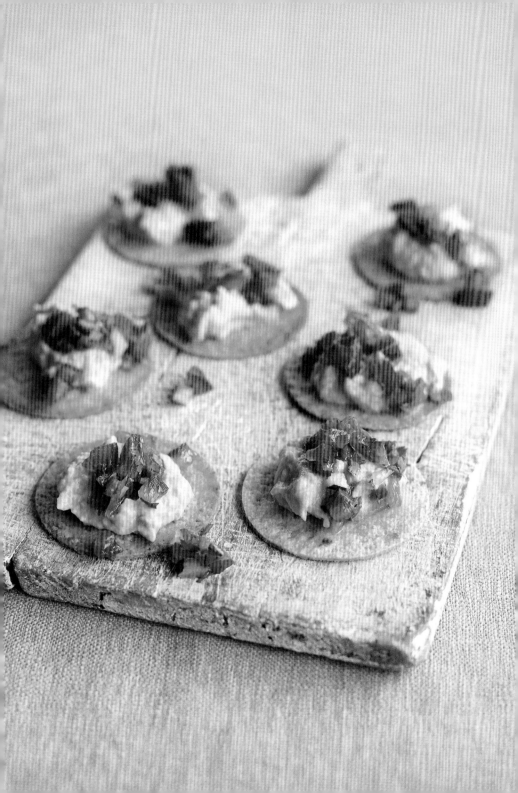

BRUSCHETTA WITH TOMATOES & BASIL

Use fresh, firm tomatoes to ensure the best antioxidant content and prepare yourself for a rejuvenating lycopene hit.

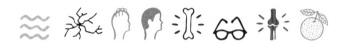

Preparation time: 10 minutes
Cooking time: 5 minutes
Serves 4

200 g (7 oz) **cherry tomatoes**, quartered
1 small **red onion**, thinly sliced
1 **garlic clove**, crushed
1 tbsp **balsamic vinegar**
3 tbsps **olive oil**
4 thick slices of **brown sourdough bread**
handful of **basil** leaves, torn
sea salt and **black pepper**

Place the tomatoes in a bowl with the onion, garlic, vinegar and half the olive oil. Season to taste, stir to combine and set aside.

Brush both sides of the bread slices with the remaining oil and place under a preheated hot grill until browned all over. Transfer to a plate and top with the tomato mixture, juice and all, and scatter the basil on top. Season with pepper and serve.

ROSEMARY OATCAKES

These oaty bites are simply delicious on their own or topped with cream cheese and a few purple-red grapes.

Preparation time: 15 minutes
Cooking time: 15 minutes
Makes 20-24

....

200 g (7 oz) **porridge oats**
leaves from 3 **rosemary sprigs**
125 g (4 oz) **wholemeal flour**,
plus extra for dusting
¾ tsp **baking powder**
pinch of **salt**
75 g (3 oz) chilled **unsalted butter**, diced
100 ml (3½ fl oz) **milk**

Place the oats and rosemary in the bowl of a food processor and blitz until they resemble breadcrumbs. Add the flour, baking powder and salt and blitz again to mix.

....

Add the butter, then process until it is mixed in. With the motor still running, pour in the milk through the feed tube until the dough forms a ball.

....

Turn the dough out onto a lightly floured surface and roll out to about 4-5 mm (¼ inch) thick. Cut out 20-24 rounds using a 5-6 cm (2-2½ inch) plain biscuit cutter, re-rolling the trimmings as necessary.

....

Arrange the cakes on a baking sheet and place in a preheated oven, 190°C (375°F), Gas Mark 5, for 12-15 minutes until golden at the edges. Transfer to a wire rack to cool. Store any leftover oatcakes in an airtight container for up to a week.

....

SPICED RAISIN & CRANBERRY COOKIES

Jewel-like cranberries are excellent for your heart, brain, skin, digestive system, kidneys and teeth, making these the perfect guilt-free snack.

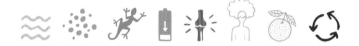

Preparation time: 10 minutes
Cooking time: 15 minutes
Makes 8
....

125 g (4 oz) **butter**
125 g (4 oz) **light muscovado sugar**
1 tbsp **honey**
125 g (4 oz) **self-raising flour**
½ tsp ground **mixed spice**
125 g (4 oz) **porridge oats**
50 g (2 oz) **raisins**
50 g (2 oz) **dried cranberries**

Place the butter, muscovado sugar and honey in a saucepan over a medium heat until just melted. Remove from the heat and stir in the flour, mixed spice, porridge oats and fruit.
....

Roll the mixture into 8 balls and arrange the balls, well spaced, on 2 lined baking sheets. Flatten them slightly and place in a preheated oven, 180°C (350°F), Gas Mark 4, for about 10–12 minutes or until golden. Cool on the baking sheets before serving. The cookies can be stored in an airtight container for up to a week.
....

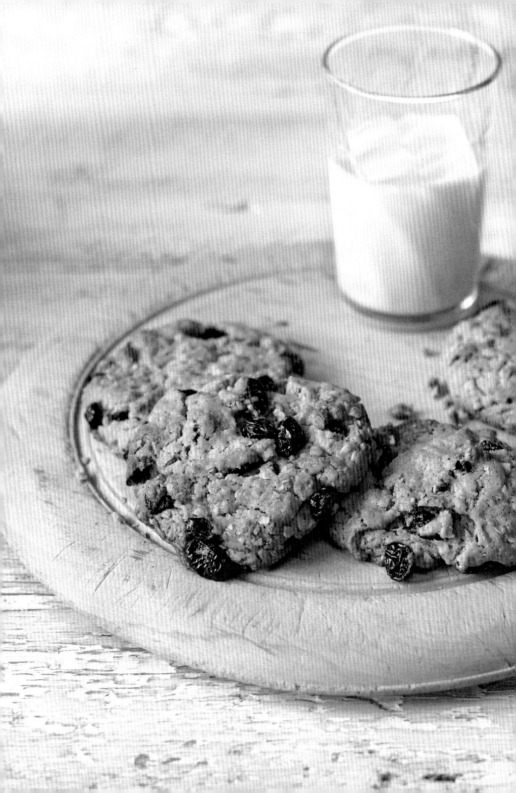

CARROT & LENTIL MUFFINS

High in fibre and full of carroty goodness, these yummy muffins are so moreish you'll never manage to stop at one.

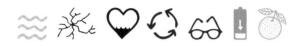

Preparation time: 10 minutes
Cooking time: 30 minutes
Makes 12
....

75 g (3 oz) split **red lentils**
275 ml (9 fl oz) **water**
275 g (9 oz) **plain wholemeal flour**
2 tbsps **ground flax seeds**
1½ tsps **baking powder**
50 g (2 oz) **dark muscovado sugar**
1 tsp **ground cinnamon**
½ tsp **ground cloves**
3 tbsps **ready-made apple sauce**
3 tbsps clear **honey**
3 tbsps **sunflower oil**
1 **egg**
1 large **carrot**, peeled and grated
2-3 tbsps **milk** or **soya milk** (optional)

Place the lentils and measurement water in a saucepan, bring to the boil and cook for about 8 minutes until tender. Drain well and allow to cool a little.

....

Place the wholemeal flour, flax seeds and baking powder in a large bowl and stir in the muscovado sugar and spices. Place the lentils in a food processor with the apple sauce, honey, oil and egg and blitz until smooth.

....

Pour the wet ingredients into the dry and gently stir with a metal spoon until only just combined, stirring in the grated carrots when nearly blended and adding a little milk to loosen the mixture, if needed. The mixture should look craggy, with specks of flour still visible.

....

Spoon the mixture into the holes of a 12-hole muffin tin lined with paper cases. Place in a preheated oven, 180°C (350°F), Gas Mark 4, for 18-20 minutes or until golden and well risen. Serve warm or cold. The muffins can be stored in an airtight container for up to 4 days and can be frozen.

....

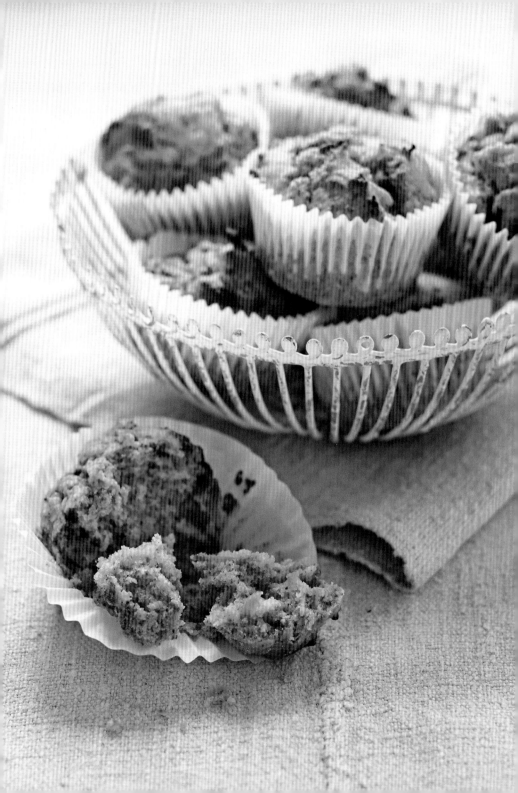

BANANA, OAT & BLACKBERRY MUFFINS

These muffins have plenty of fibre and a host of antioxidants and omega oils to encourage wellbeing on all levels.

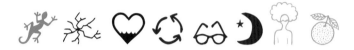

Preparation time: 15 minutes
Cooking time: 20 minutes
Makes 12
················

300 g (10 oz) **self-raising flour**
1 tsp **bicarbonate of soda**
100 g (3½ oz) **muscovado sugar**
75 g (3 oz) **pinhead oatmeal**
2 ripe **bananas**, peeled
275 ml (9 fl oz) **live natural yogurt**
75 ml (3 fl oz) **olive oil**
2 **eggs**, lightly beaten
150 g (5 oz) **blackberries**
1 tsp **ground cinnamon**
1 tsp **golden granulated sugar**

Sift into a large bowl the flour, bicarbonate of soda and sugar and stir in the oatmeal. Mash together the bananas, yogurt, olive oil and eggs in a separate bowl and stir until well blended and fairly smooth.
················

Next fold the banana mixture into the flour mixture and gently stir with a metal spoon until only just combined. The mixture should look craggy, with specks of flour still visible. Add the blackberries and stir once or twice so they are mixed in but not crushed.
················

Spoon the mixture into a 12-hole muffin tin lined with paper cases. Mix the cinnamon and granulated sugar together and sprinkle over the tops of the muffins.
················

Place in a preheated oven, 180°C (350°F), Gas Mark 4, for about 20 minutes or until golden and well risen. Serve warm or cold. The muffins can be stored in an airtight container for up to 4 days and are suitable for freezing.
················

CRANBERRY MUFFINS

Light and fluffy, these scrumptious muffins contain antioxidant-rich cranberries and flavonoid-rich chocolate.

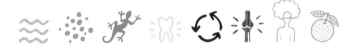

Preparation time: 10 minutes
Cooking time: 20 minutes
Makes 12

....

150 g (5 oz) **plain flour**
150 g (5 oz) **self-raising flour**
1 tbsp **baking powder**
65 g (2½ oz) **light muscovado sugar**
50 g (2 oz) **stem ginger in syrup**,
drained and finely chopped
100 g (3½ oz) **dried cranberries**
100 g (3½ oz) **dark chocolate chips**
1 **egg**
250 ml (8 fl oz) **skimmed milk** or **soya milk**
4 tbsps **vegetable oil**

Sift both the flours and baking powder into a large bowl, then stir in the sugar, ginger, cranberries and dark chocolate chips until evenly distributed. Beat together the egg, milk and oil in a separate bowl, then add the resulting liquid to the flour mixture and stir gently with a metal spoon until just combined. The mixture should look craggy, with specks of flour still visible.

....

Line a 12-hole muffin tin with paper cases and spoon the mixture into them. Place in a preheated oven, 200°C (400°F), Gas Mark 6, for about 18–20 minutes or until golden and well risen. Serve slightly warm. The muffins can be stored in an airtight container for up to 4 days and can be frozen.

....

AUBERGINE & SESAME NOODLE SALAD

This Chinese-inspired dish is delicious whether hot or cold, making it ideal for a lunch box. It has the rejuvenating power of aubergines to boot!

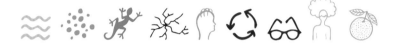

Preparation time: 25 minutes
Cooking time: 30 minutes
Serves 4

2 **aubergines**
1 tsp **chilli oil**
4 tbsps **sesame oil**
6 tbsps **light soy sauce**
4 tbsps **sweet chilli sauce**
2 tbsps **rice wine**
3 tbsps **clear honey**
3 tbsps **sesame seeds**, toasted
150 g (5 oz) dried fine **egg noodles**
1 tsp finely chopped fresh **root ginger**
1 **garlic clove**, crushed
25 g (1 oz) **baby spinach**
1 **red pepper**, cored, deseeded and finely chopped
8 **spring onions**, thinly sliced
50 g (2 oz) **bean sprouts**
large handful of **coriander** leaves, roughly chopped

Place the whole aubergines on a baking sheet, prick all over with a fork and cook in a preheated oven, 200°C (400°F), Gas Mark 6, for 30 minutes until tender.

Meanwhile, mix together the oils, soy sauce, chilli sauce, rice wine and honey in a bowl. Stir in the toasted sesame seeds and divide the dressing between 2 wide bowls.

Cook the noodles in a saucepan of boiling water according to packet instructions until just tender. Drain, place in one of the bowls of dressing and toss to coat evenly. Mix the ginger and garlic into the other bowl of dressing.

Cut the aubergines in half lengthways and use a spoon to scoop the flesh into the bowl of garlicky dressing. Stir in the spinach, red pepper, spring onions and bean sprouts, then add the dressed noodles and toss to mix well. Scatter with the coriander and serve warm or cold.

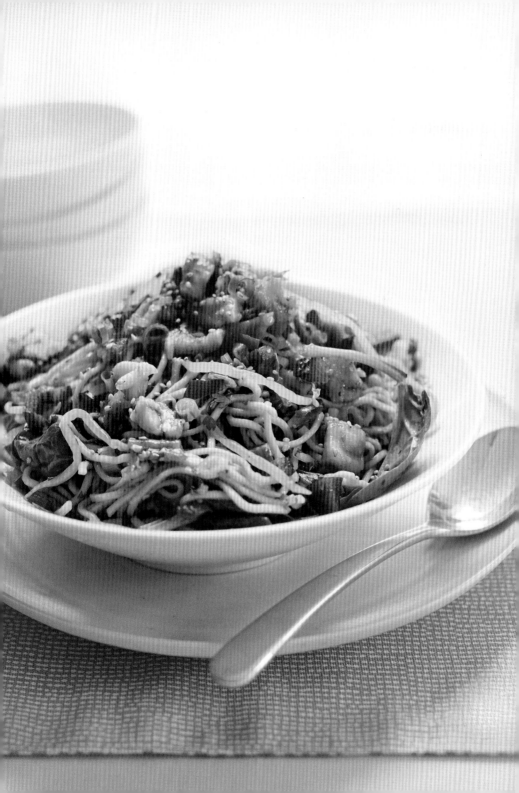

AVOCADO & SARDINE SALAD WITH ZESTY DRESSING

This tangy, fragrant salad offers a burst of protein, omega-3 oils, healthy fats and vitamin E to stop ageing in its tracks.

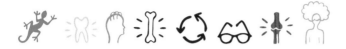

Preparation time: 15 minutes
Serves 4
....

2 x 125 g (4 oz) cans **sardine fillets**
in olive oil, drained
handful of fresh **coriander**, finely chopped,
plus extra to serve
1 **celery** stick, finely chopped
1 **spring onion**, chopped
2 tbsps good-quality **mayonnaise**
finely grated rind and juice of 1 **lime**
3 handfuls of mixed **salad leaves**
2 **avocados**, peeled, pitted
and cut into wedges
sea salt and **black pepper**

Dressing
finely grated rind and juice of 1 **lime**
2 tbsps **extra virgin olive oil**
½ tsp **sea salt**
½ tsp **sugar**
2 tbsps finely chopped fresh **coriander**
1 tbsp **coconut cream**

Place the sardines, coriander, celery, spring onion, mayonnaise, lime rind and juice in a large bowl, season to taste and toss together. Whisk together the dressing ingredients in a separate bowl.
....

Arrange the salad leaves on a large plate and scatter the avocado wedges on top. Place the sardine mixture in a mound in the centre and drizzle over the dressing. Sprinkle with a few extra coriander leaves and a good grating of pepper and serve immediately.
....

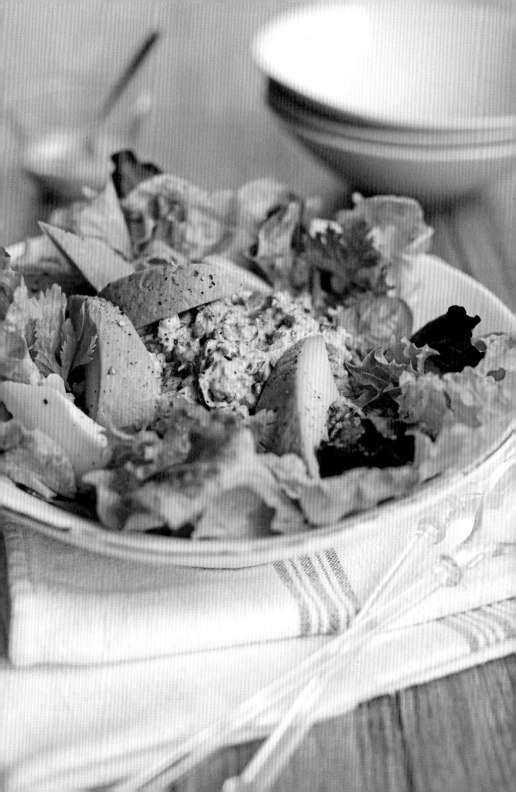

FENNEL & CUMIN WALDORF SALAD

A twist on the world-famous salad created at New York City's Waldorf Hotel, this one benefits from all the super-nutrients of fabulous fennel.

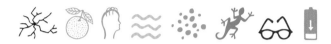

Preparation time: 10 minutes
Cooking time: 5 minutes
Serves 4
....

60 g (2¼ oz) **walnut pieces**
1 tsp **ground cumin**
300 g (10 oz) **live natural yogurt**
100 g (3½ oz) **green** and **black grapes**, halved
1 small **fennel bulb**, thinly sliced
6 **celery** sticks, diagonally sliced
1 **green apple**, cored, quartered and thinly sliced
60 g (2¼ oz) **sultanas**
sea salt and **black pepper**

Heat a nonstick frying pan over a medium-low heat and dry-fry the walnut pieces for 3–4 minutes, stirring frequently, until lightly golden. Leave to cool slightly.
....

Place the cumin and live yogurt in a large bowl, season to taste and mix well. Add all the remaining ingredients, including the toasted walnuts, and toss in the dressing until well coated. Either serve immediately or cover and chill until required.
....

CARROT & PUY LENTIL SALAD

With plenty of antioxidants, protein, B vitamins and fibre, this surprisingly sweet salad is a great choice to form the mainstay of any anti-ageing diet!

Preparation time: 15 minutes, plus cooling
Cooking time: 35 minutes
Serves 4

....

500 g (1 lb) **carrots**, scrubbed
1 tbsp **olive oil**
1 tbsp **cumin seeds**
1 tsp **dried thyme**
1 tbsp clear **honey**
400 g (13 oz) can **Puy lentils**, rinsed and drained
1 large **red onion**, finely chopped
60 ml (2½ fl oz) **cider vinegar**
1 tbsp **hazelnut oil**
large handful of **mint** leaves, chopped
100 g (3½ oz) **rocket** or **watercress**
25 g (1 oz) **hazelnuts**, toasted
100 g (3½ oz) **feta cheese**
sea salt and **black pepper**

Cut the scrubbed carrots into matchsticks and place in a roasting tin with the olive oil, cumin and thyme. Place in a preheated oven, 180°C (350°F), Gas Mark 4, for 30 minutes, turning frequently. Drizzle all over with the honey and return to the oven for a further 5 minutes, then allow to cool.

Meanwhile, place the lentils, onion, vinegar and hazelnut oil in a large saucepan, season to taste and heat through gently, stirring frequently. Remove from the heat and allow to cool, then stir in the mint.

To serve, arrange the rocket on a large plate, top with the lentils then the carrots. Scatter with toasted hazelnuts and then crumble over the feta cheese. Grind some pepper over the top and serve.

BROCCOLI SALAD WITH DILL & PINE NUTS

This hearty raw broccoli and fruit salad provides loads of fibre and antioxidants to help turn back the clock.

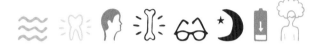

Preparation time: 15 minutes, plus standing
Serves 4
....

2 large heads of **broccoli**,
cut into tiny florets
handful of **watercress**, torn
1 **red onion**, finely sliced
100 g (3½ oz) **grapes**, quartered
100 g (3½ oz) **blackberries**, halved
100 g (3½ oz) **dried cranberries**, halved
25 g (1 oz) **pomegranate seeds**
50 g (2 oz) **pine nuts**, toasted

Dressing
2 tbsps good-quality **mayonnaise**
2 tbsps **live natural yogurt**
finely grated rind and juice of 1 **lemon**
2 tbsps finely chopped **dill**
sea salt and **black pepper**

Place the broccoli, heads watercress, onion, quartered grapes, blackberries, cranberries, pomegranate seeds and pine nuts in a large bowl and toss together.

....

Place all the dressing ingredients in a small bowl, season to taste and whisk to combine. Pour over the salad and gently toss to coat. Set aside for 10 minutes before serving to allow the flavours to mingle. Any leftover salad can be stored in an airtight container in the refrigerator for 2–3 days.

....

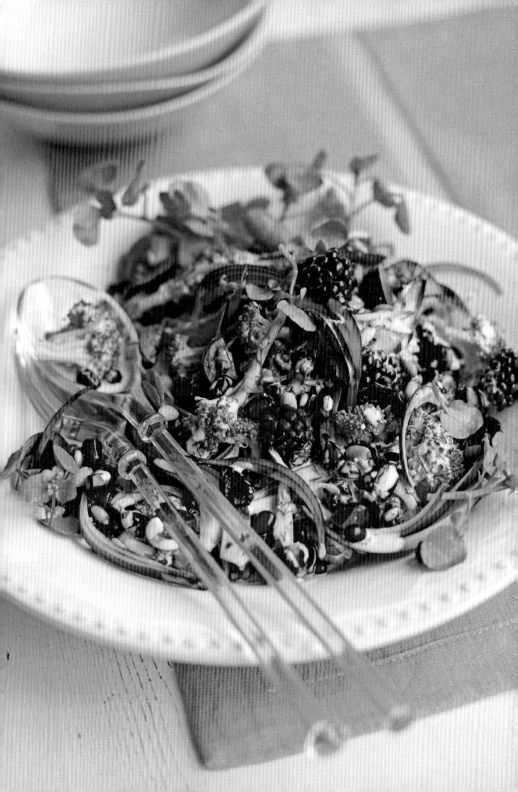

CARROT & BEETROOT TABBOULEH

A delicious Middle Eastern salad custom-designed to enhance youthfulness, with its wide range of age-defying nutrients.

Preparation time: 20 minutes
Cooking time: 20 minutes
Serves 4

150 g (5 oz) **bulgar wheat**
1 **garlic clove**, crushed
pinch of **ground cinnamon**
pinch of **ground allspice**
2 tbsps **pomegranate molasses**
5 tbsps **extra virgin olive oil**
1 **carrot**, grated
125 g (4 oz) **cooked beetroot**, cubed
2 **spring onions**, sliced
½ **green chilli**, chopped
large handful of **mint**, chopped
large handful of **parsley**, chopped
50 g (2 oz) **feta cheese**
25 g (1 oz) **pomegranate seeds**
sea salt and **black pepper**

Cook the bulgar wheat in a saucepan of lightly salted water according to packet instructions until tender. Drain thoroughly.

Place the garlic clove, spices, pomegranate molasses and olive oil in a large bowl and mix together well. Add the bulgar wheat, grated carrot, beetroot, spring onions, chilli, mint and parsley, season to taste and toss well to mix.

Arrange the salad in a serving dish, scatter the feta and pomegranate seeds over the top and serve.

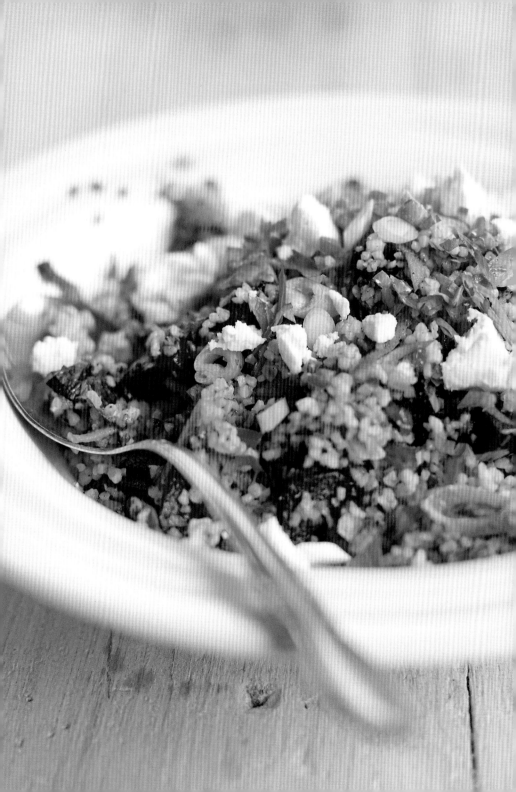

PESTO BROCCOLI WITH POACHED EGGS

This sensational lunch dish ticks all the boxes when it comes to anti-ageing vitamins and minerals, and it's satisfyingly tasty.

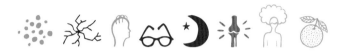

Preparation time: 10 minutes
Cooking time: 10 minutes
Serves 4
....

625 g (1¼ lb) **broccoli** florets
300 g (10 oz) **sugar snap peas**
1 tsp **vinegar**
4 **eggs**
75 g (3 oz) **sun-dried tomatoes**, chopped
sea salt and **black pepper**
Parmesan cheese shavings, to serve

Pesto
10 g (3/8 oz) **basil** leaves
5 g (¼ oz) toasted **pine nuts**
5 g (¼ oz) **Parmesan cheese**, grated
1 small **garlic clove**, crushed
15–20 ml (½–¾ fl oz) **olive oil**

For the pesto, place the basil and pine nuts in a mini processor and blitz until broken down. Add the cheese and garlic and blitz briefly. With the motor still running, slowly pour in the oil through the feed tube until combined. Season to taste.
....

Cook the broccoli florets and peas in a large saucepan of lightly salted boiling water for about 7–8 minutes or until softened but still a little crunchy.
....

Meanwhile, bring a saucepan of water to the boil and add the vinegar. Reduce the heat to a very low simmer and break the eggs gently into the water. Cook for about 5 minutes or until the whites are cooked through and the yolks are still runny.
....

Drain the vegetables, then return to the pan and stir in 1½ tablespoons of the pesto (any remaining pesto can be stored in an airtight container in the refrigerator). Add the sun-dried tomatoes and gently toss together until well coated.
....

Divide the vegetables between 4 plates, top with the eggs and Parmesan shavings and sprinkle with pepper to taste before serving.
....

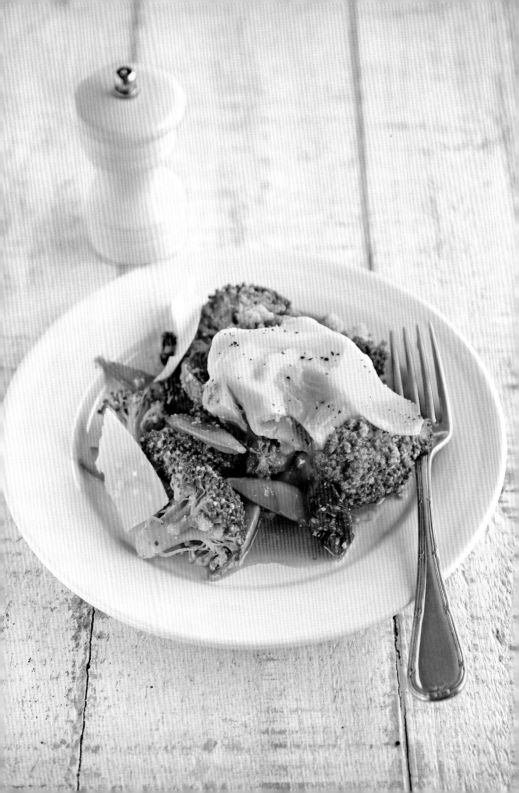

MEDITERRANEAN STUFFED PEPPERS

These easy-to-prepare stuffed peppers are chock-full of protein, antioxidants, amino acids, calcium and omega oils to support health on all levels.

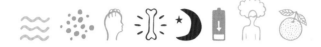

Preparation time: 15 minutes
Cooking time: 40 minutes
Serves 4

100 g (3½ oz) **quinoa**
12 **sunblush tomatoes**, sliced,
plus 2 tbsps oil from the jar
1 small **onion**, finely chopped
2 **garlic cloves**, crushed
1 tsp **dried oregano**
1 tsp **dried thyme**
1 tbsp **balsamic vinegar**
12 **black olives**, sliced
100 g (3½ oz) **feta cheese**, cubed
handful of **basil** leaves, torn
4 large **red peppers**
sea salt and **black pepper**
green salad, to serve

Cook the quinoa in a large saucepan of lightly salted boiling water according to packet instructions, until tender.

Meanwhile, heat the sunblush tomato oil in a large saucepan or wok over a medium heat, add the onion, garlic, oregano and thyme and cook for 5–10 minutes until the onion is soft.

Stir in the quinoa, balsamic vinegar, black olives and sunblush tomatoes, then cook for a further 2–3 minutes. Remove from the heat, season to taste, then stir in the feta and basil.

Slice the tops off the peppers, retaining the lids but removing the cores and seeds. Spoon the quinoa mixture into the peppers, replace the lids and arrange in an ovenproof dish. Cook the peppers in a preheated oven, 180°C (350°F), Gas Mark 4, for 20–25 minutes until the peppers have softened but still have a little bite. Serve hot or cold with a green salad.

GAZPACHO

The tasty garnish makes this superfood-rich Spanish soup into a fabulous meal in a bowl.

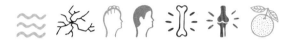

Preparation time: 15 minutes
Cooking time: 5 minutes
Serves 4

....

4 **red peppers**, cored, deseeded and roughly chopped
1 **red onion**, roughly chopped
2 **cucumbers**, roughly chopped
handful of **basil** leaves
handful of **parsley** leaves
2 **garlic cloves**, peeled
2 tbsps **sherry vinegar** or **balsamic vinegar**
150 ml (¼ pint) **olive oil**
450 ml (¾ pint) chilled **tomato juice**
sea salt and **black pepper**

Croûtons
1 tbsp **butter**, melted
1 tbsp **olive oil**
1 **garlic clove**, crushed
2 thick slices of **wholegrain bread**

To serve
1 **avocado**, peeled, pitted and diced
4 soft-boiled **eggs**, quartered

Place the vegetables, herbs and garlic in a food processor and blitz until very finely chopped. Add the vinegar, oil and tomato juice, season to taste and process again briefly. Cover and chill for about 5 minutes.

....

For the croûtons, mix the melted butter, oil and garlic in a small bowl then spread the mixture on both sides of the bread. Cut the bread into 2.5 cm (1 inch) squares.

....

Heat a large frying pan over a medium heat, add the bread squares and cook for about 5 minutes, tossing and stirring, until golden and crispy. Drain the croûtons on a sheet of kitchen paper.

....

Serve the soup in bowls topped with the croûtons, diced avocado and egg quarters.

....

ROASTED CHILLI & LEMON SARDINES

An intense lemon flavour, a kick of chilli and all the omega goodness of sardines make this pure youth food on a plate.

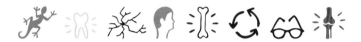

Preparation time: 10 minutes
Cooking time: 15 minutes
Serves 4

3 **garlic cloves**, finely sliced
2 **red chillies**, deseeded and finely sliced
finely sliced rind of 1 **preserved lemon**
3 tbsps **argan oil** or **olive oil**
juice of 1 **lemon**
8 **sardines**, gutted and cleaned
sea salt and **black pepper**
small bunch of **flat leaf parsley**, finely chopped, to garnish
wholegrain crusty bread, to serve

Mix the garlic, chillies and preserved lemon rind in a bowl, then add the oil and lemon juice and season well.

Spread some of the mixture over the base of an ovenproof dish. Arrange the sardines on top of the mixture in a single layer and spoon the remaining mixture on top. Place them in a preheated oven, 200°C (400°F), Gas Mark 6, for 10–15 minutes, or until the sardines are cooked through.

Transfer to a serving dish, spoon over the juices and garnish with the parsley. Serve with wholegrain crusty bread.

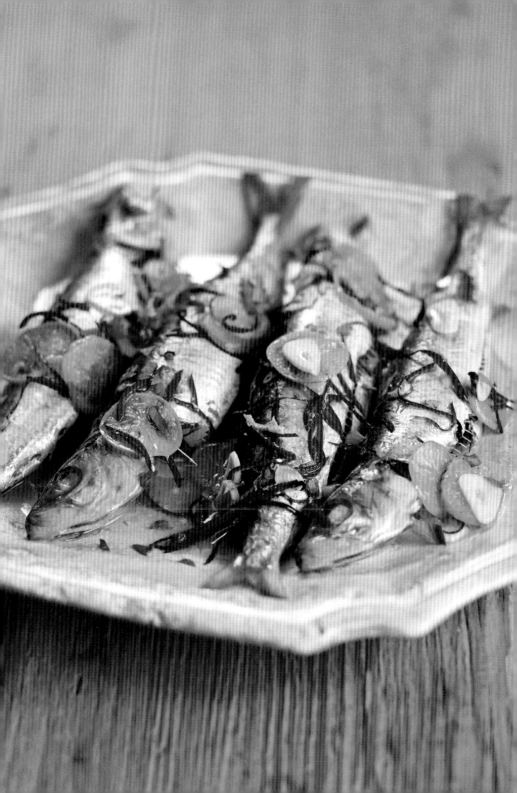

FENNEL & MUSHROOM TARTS

These luxurious little tarts are packed with protein, fibre and a wealth of vitamins and minerals to give you a healthy glow.

Preparation time: 15 minutes
Cooking time: 40 minutes
Serves 4
················

250 g (8 oz) **ready-made shortcrust pastry**
flour, for dusting
75 g (3 oz) grated **Parmesan cheese**
1 tbsp **olive oil**
3 **garlic cloves**, crushed
1 small **red onion**, very finely chopped
1 tsp **dried thyme**
175 g (6 oz) mixed **mushrooms**
1 **fennel bulb**, thinly sliced
3 **eggs**, lightly beaten
50 g (2 oz) **Emmental cheese**
handful of **parsley**, chopped
sea salt and **black pepper**
leafy **green salad**, to serve

Roll out the ready-made shortcut pastry on a lightly floured surface to roughly 3 mm (⅛ inch) thick, and use it to line 4 greased 10 cm (4 inch) tartlet tins. Gently rub one-third of the Parmesan cheese into the lined pastry cases and chill in the refrigerator for 10 minutes.

················

Heat the olive oil in a large frying pan over a medium heat and add the garlic, onion and thyme. Cook for 5 minutes until starting to soften, then add the mushrooms and fennel. Cook for a further 5 minutes, then remove from the heat.

················

Place the eggs in a bowl with the Emmental, the remaining Parmesan and the chopped parsley, season to taste and beat together.

················

Use a slotted spoon to divide the mushroom and fennel mixture between the pastry cases and place them on a baking sheet. Pour the egg mixture into the tartlets and place in a preheated oven, 180°C (350°F), Gas Mark 4, for 30 minutes or until the egg mixture has set. Serve either warm or cold with a leafy green salad.

················

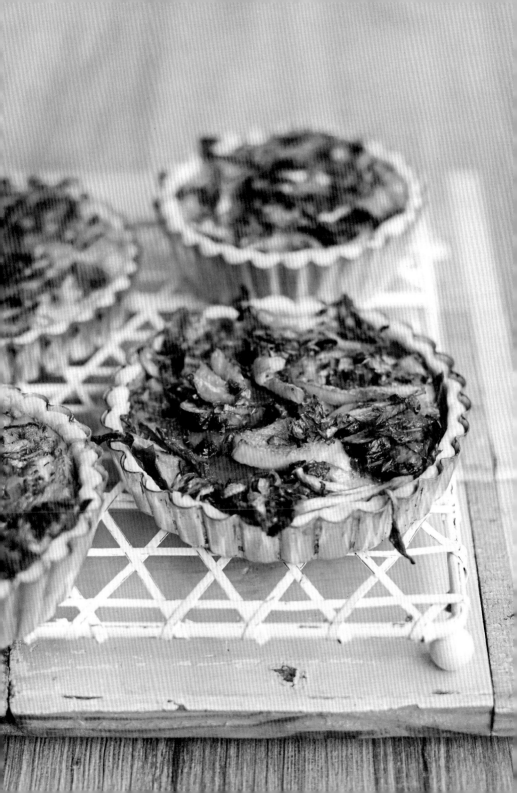

WATERCRESS SOUP WITH CHEESY OATCAKES

This calcium- and antioxidant-rich soup can be served warm or cold. The oatcakes will help to keep blood sugar levels steady.

Preparation time: 30 minutes
Cooking time: 30 minutes
Serves 4

....

1 tbsp **olive oil**
3 large **potatoes**,
peeled and cut into chunks
2 **onions**, chopped
1 **garlic clove**, chopped
600 ml (1 pint) **vegetable** or **chicken stock**
4 large bunches of **watercress**, rinsed
and chopped, plus extra, to garnish
finely grated rind and juice of 1 **lemon**
sea salt and **black pepper**
3 tbsp **live Greek yogurt**, to serve

Cheesy oatcakes
125 g (4 oz) **oatmeal**
150 g (5 oz) **porridge oats**
75 g (3 oz) **mature Cheddar cheese**, grated
60 ml (2½ fl oz) **olive oil**
90 ml (3¼ fl oz) hot **water**
flour, for dusting

Place the oatmeal and porridge oats in a bowl and season. Stir in the Cheddar and then the oil. Slowly add the measurement hot water, using a fork to combine, until you have a firm dough. Then turn the dough out on an oiled surface and knead it until well combined. Add a little more water if needed.

Roll out on a lightly floured surface to about 3 mm (⅛ inch) thick. Cut into squares with a knife or cut out rounds with a pastry cutter. Transfer to 2 lined baking sheets and put in a preheated oven, 180°C (350°F), Gas Mark 4, for 20 minutes. Turn the oatcakes over and bake for a further 10 minutes. Remove from the oven and set aside to cool.

Meanwhile, heat the oil in a large saucepan over a medium heat and add the potatoes, onions and garlic. Cook for about 5 minutes, stirring constantly, until the onions are soft. Add the stock and bring to the boil. Reduce the heat and simmer for about 20 minutes until the potatoes are soft.

Stir in the watercress, lemon rind and juice and season to taste. Cook for a further 2–3 minutes, then remove from the heat. Purée until smooth. Top each portion with a swirl of Greek yogurt, a sprig of watercress and a grating of pepper and serve with the oatcakes.

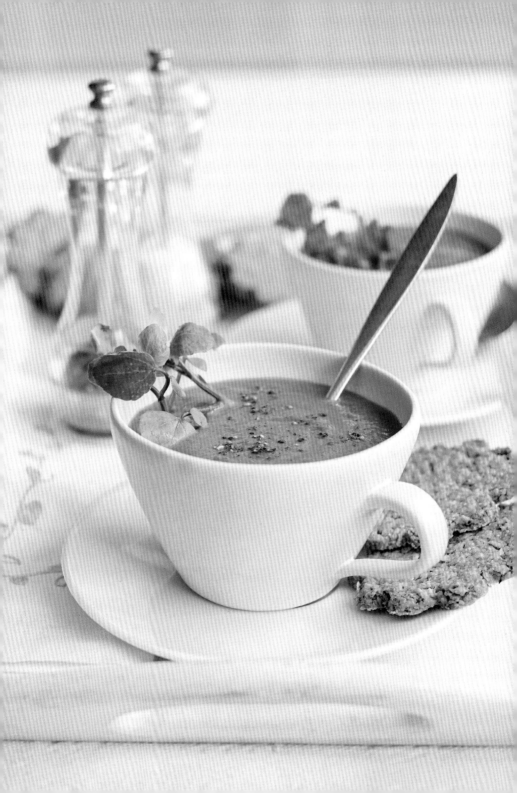

CHILLED AVOCADO SOUP

A sophisticated soup full of omega-3s and anti-ageing vitamins A, C, E and K, as well as heart-healthy potassium.

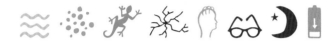

Preparation time: 10 minutes
Serves 4
················

3 ripe **avocados**, peeled, pitted and diced
1 small **red onion**, roughly chopped
3–4 drops of **Tabasco sauce**
3 tbsps **lime juice**
600 ml (1 pint) **buttermilk**
4 tbsps chopped fresh **coriander**
12 **ice cubes**
wholewheat tortillas, warmed
and cut into strips, to serve

Place most of the avocado pieces in a food processor, reserving a handful for garnish, with the remaining ingredients except the ice cubes and blend until smooth.
··

Divide evenly between 4 serving bowls and top each portion with 3 ice cubes and some of the reserved avocado. Serve immediately with warmed tortilla strips.
··

CARROT, CORIANDER & LENTIL SOUP

Hormone-balancing carrots combine with high-fibre lentils and fragrant coriander to make this rich, filling soup.

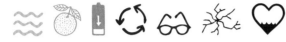

Preparation time: 10 minutes
Cooking time: 30 minutes
Serves 4
....

2 tbsps **argan oil** or **olive oil**
1 **onion**, finely chopped
25 g (1 oz) fresh **root ginger**, chopped
2–3 **garlic cloves**, finely chopped
2 tsps **coriander seeds**
1 tsp **cumin seeds**
1 tsp **granulated sugar**
4 **carrots**, peeled and diced
150 g (5 oz) **brown lentils**, rinsed
1–2 tsps **ras el hanout spice mix**
400 g (13 oz) can **chopped tomatoes**, drained of juice
1.2 litres (2 pints) hot **chicken stock**
bunch of fresh **coriander**, finely chopped
sea salt and **black pepper**

To serve
3–4 tbsps **live natural yogurt**
crusty wholegrain bread

Heat the oil in a heavy-based saucepan over a medium heat, stir in the onion, root ginger, garlic cloves, seeds and sugar and cook for 2–3 minutes. Add the diced carrots and cook for 2 minutes, stirring to coat well. Stir in the lentils, ras el hanout spice mix, tomatoes and stock and bring to the boil, then reduce the heat and simmer for 20 minutes.

....

Season the soup to taste and stir in most of the chopped coriander, reserving a little for garnish, then cook for a further 5 minutes or until the carrots and lentils are tender. Swirl a little of the live yogurt into the soup, then divide between 4 bowls. Garnish with the remaining coriander and yogurt and serve with crusty bread.

....

CHICKEN MOLE

This rich Mexican chicken and chocolate dish is a treat – and it's chock-full of powerful anti-ageing nutrients.

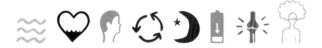

Preparation time: 25 minutes
Cooking time: 1½ hours
Serves 4
....

3 tbsps **vegetable oil**
1 oven-ready **chicken**,
about 1.5 kg (3 lb), jointed
1 **onion**, chopped
1 **green pepper**, cored,
deseeded and chopped
½ tsp **ground allspice**
½ tsp **ground cinnamon**
½ tsp **ground cumin**
1 tsp **chilli powder**
2 **garlic cloves**, crushed
200 g (7 oz) can **chopped tomatoes**
300 ml (½ pint) **chicken stock**
25 g (1 oz) soft **corn tortilla**,
plus extra to serve
40 g (1½ oz) **blanched almonds**,
roughly chopped
2 tbsps **sesame seeds**,
plus extra for sprinkling
15 g (½ oz) **plain dark chocolate**
(85 per cent cocoa solids),
roughly chopped
sea salt and **black pepper**
chopped fresh **coriander**, to garnish

Heat the oil in a flameproof casserole and fry the chicken pieces for 5 minutes until golden on all sides. Transfer to a plate. Add the onion and green pepper to the casserole and fry gently for 5 minutes until softened, stirring in the spices and garlic for the last few minutes.

....

Add the tomatoes and half the stock and bring to the boil. Return the chicken to the casserole, cover and place in a preheated oven, 180°C (350°F), Gas Mark 4, for 45 minutes.

....

Meanwhile, tear the tortilla into pieces and place in a food processor with the almonds and sesame seeds. Blitz until finely ground. Add the remaining stock and process again until smooth. Stir the almond mixture and chocolate into the casserole and return to the oven for a further 30 minutes until the chicken is cooked through and tender.

....

Season to taste, sprinkle with extra sesame seeds and scatter with the coriander. Serve with warmed tortillas.

....

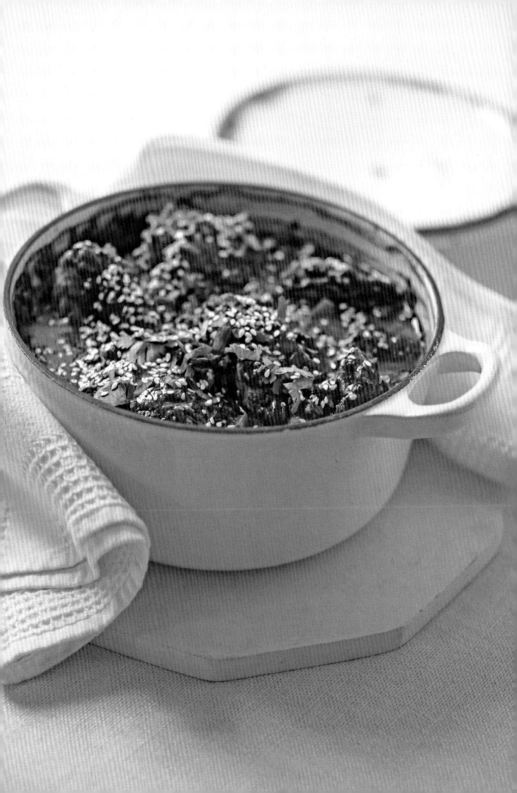

FENNEL-ROASTED LAMB WITH FIGS

Impressive enough for any dinner party, this has a cornucopia of vitamins and minerals to protect the body both inside and out.

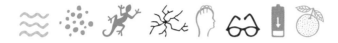

Preparation time: 15 minutes
Cooking time: 25 minutes
Serves 4
....

3 **garlic cloves**, chopped
25 g (1 oz) fresh **root ginger**,
peeled and chopped
1 **red chilli**, deseeded and chopped
1 tsp **sea salt**
1 tsp ground **coriander**
1 tsp **ground cumin**
2 tbsps **smen, ghee** or **softened butter**
2 tsps **fennel seeds**
700 g (1 lb 6 oz) piece of lean **lamb**
fillet or loin
1 **fennel bulb**, sliced
4 fresh **figs**, halved or quartered
2 tbsps clear **honey**
black pepper
small bunch of fresh coriander,
finely chopped, to garnish
couscous, to serve (optional)

Using a pestle and mortar, pound the garlic, ginger, chilli and salt to form a coarse paste, then add the ground spices. Beat the paste into the smen, ghee or butter with the fennel seeds.

....

Cut small incisions in the lamb and rub the mixture all over the meat, pressing it into the incisions. Place the lamb and fennel in a roasting tin and place in a preheated oven, 200°C (400°F), Gas Mark 6, for 15 minutes.

....

Baste with the cooking juices, arrange the figs around the lamb and drizzle with the honey. Season to taste, then return to the oven and cook for a further 10 minutes until cooked through. Garnish with the chopped fresh coriander and serve thickly sliced, with couscous, if liked.

....

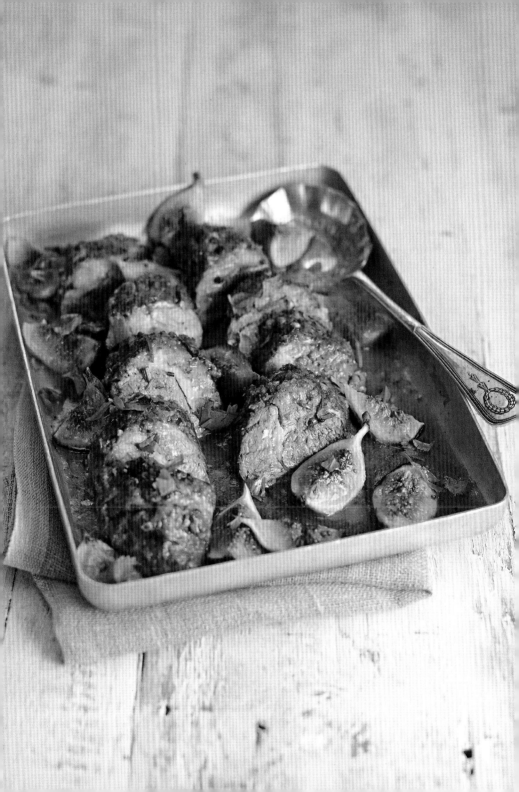

GUAVA-GLAZED PORK TENDERLOIN

Simply bursting with fruity, spicy flavour, this rejuvenating dish is full of powerful antioxidants to support your skin, bones, eyes, teeth, heart and blood vessels.

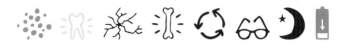

Preparation time: 15 minutes, plus resting
Cooking time: 50 minutes
Serves 4

1 kg (2 lb) piece of **pork tenderloin**
finely grated rind and juice of 1 **lime**
1 tbsp **olive oil**
1 tsp clear **honey**
200 g (7 oz) mixed **herbs** and **salad leaves**
50 g (2 oz) **pomegranate seeds**
sea salt and **black pepper**

Guava glaze
1 tbsp **olive oil**
1 small **onion**, finely chopped
1 **garlic clove**, crushed
1 small **red chilli**, deseeded
and finely chopped
1 tbsp **paprika**
2 tsps **ground coriander**
1 tsp **ground cinnamon**
1 tsp **ground ginger**
2 tsps **sea salt**
125 ml (4 fl oz) **guava juice**
finely grated rind and juice of 1 large **orange**
1 **guava**, peeled, deseeded and diced
1 tbsp **cider vinegar**

For the glaze, heat the oil in a saucepan over a low heat, add the onion, garlic cloved and chopped chilli and cook for 5–10 minutes or until the onion is soft. Add all the remaining glaze ingredients, bring the glaze to the boil then reduce the temperature and simmer for 20 minutes, stirring constantly, until the guava breaks down and the sauce begins to thicken. Remove from the heat and brush half of the glaze over the pork tenderloin.

Transfer to a baking sheet and place in a preheated oven, 180°C (350°F), Gas Mark 4, for 10 minutes. Brush with a little more of the glaze and return to the oven for 10 minutes, until just cooked through. Remove from the oven, pour over the remaining glaze, cover lightly with foil and rest for 10 minutes.

Whisk together the lime juice and rind, olive oil and honey and season to taste. Sprinkle over the herbs and salad leaves, toss gently, and scatter the pomegranate seeds over the top. Slice the pork and serve with the salad.

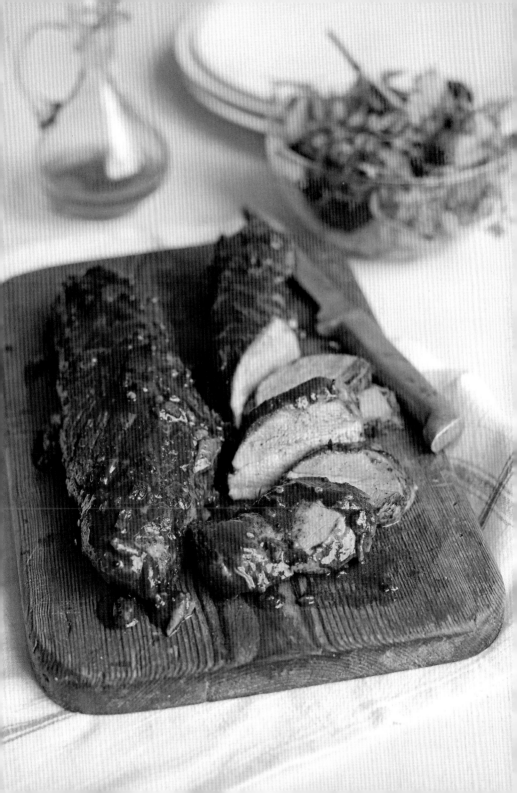

TOASTED QUINOA, TUNA & LENTIL SALAD

This delicious, savoury and satisfying salad is rich in omega-3 oils, protein, fibre and antioxidants.

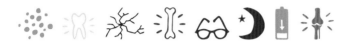

Preparation time: 20 minutes
Cooking time: 45 minutes
Serves 4
....

150 g (5 oz) **quinoa**, rinsed and drained
2 tbsps **olive oil**
425 ml (14½ fl oz) **vegetable stock**
150 g (5 oz) **purple sprouting broccoli**, sliced
150 g (5 oz) **asparagus** tips
150 g (5 oz) fresh **peas**
150 g (5 oz) **spring greens**, shredded
1 small **red chilli**, finely chopped
finely grated rind and juice of ½ **lemon**
1 **garlic clove**, crushed
4 fresh **tuna steaks**
400 g (13 oz) can **Puy lentils**, rinsed and drained
8 **spring onions**, diagonally sliced
handful of **mint** leaves, chopped
handful of **parsley**, chopped
3 tbsps chopped **tarragon**
sea salt and **black pepper**

Dressing
finely grated rind and juice of 1 **lemon**
2 tbsps **olive oil**
1 tsp **dried tarragon**
1 **garlic clove**, crushed

Place the rinsed quinoa in a large, nonstick saucepan over a medium heat and stir until the water evaporates. Add half the olive oil and continue stirring for about 15 minutes until the quinoa begins to brown and pop. Add the stock and bring to the boil, then reduce the heat and simmer for 20 minutes or until all the liquid has been absorbed and the quinoa is tender. Transfer to a large bowl and leave to cool.

....

Cook the broccoli, asparagus tips, peas and spring greens in a large saucepan of lightly salted boiling water for 2-3 minutes, then drain and plunge into cold water. Drain and set aside. Make the dressing by whisking all the ingredients together in a small bowl.

....

Mix the chilli, lemon rind and juice and garlic in a small bowl and rub the mixture all over the tuna steaks. Season to taste and place under a preheated hot grill for 3 minutes on each side then transfer to a chopping board.

....

Toss the blanched vegetables, lentils, spring onions and herbs with the quinoa, stir in the dressing and fluff up with a fork. Cut the tuna steaks into strips and lay on top of the salad, grind a little pepper over the top and serve.

....

ASPARAGUS & PEA QUINOA RISOTTO

Who says risotto needs rice? Protein-rich quinoa makes this a nutritious dish to preserve youthfulness and boost your health on all levels.

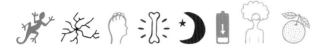

Preparation time: 5 minutes
Cooking time: 15–20 minutes
Serves 4

....

275 g (9 oz) **quinoa**, rinsed
600 ml (1 pint) hot **vegetable stock**
200 g (7 oz) frozen **peas**
200 g (7 oz) **asparagus**, chopped
1 tbsp chopped **mint**
3 tbsps grated **Parmesan cheese**
sea salt and **black pepper**

Put the quinoa and stock in a large saucepan over a high heat and bring to the boil. Then reduce the heat and simmer for 15 minutes or until the quinoa is tender, adding the peas and asparagus about 2 minutes before the end of the cooking time.

....

Drain off the excess stock, then add the mint and two-thirds of the Parmesan. Season to taste and mix well. Serve sprinkled with the remaining Parmesan.

....

MISO AUBERGINES WITH RICE NOODLES

Deep purple aubergines are a powerful source of age-busting vitamins and minerals to nourish you inside and out – brain, bones, skin, hair and eyes.

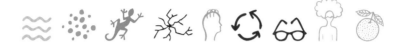

Preparation time: 10 minutes
Cooking time: 15 minutes
Serves 4
....

12 baby **aubergines**, halved
4 tbsps white **miso paste**
3 tbsps **rice wine vinegar**
2 tbsps **caster sugar**
1 tbsp **sake** or **water**
1 tbsp **sesame seeds**
125 g (4 oz) **edamame beans** (soya)
300 g (10 oz) cooked **rice noodles**
½ **cucumber**, thinly sliced
2 **spring onions**, thinly sliced
sea salt

Use a sharp knife to cut a criss-cross pattern on the cut sides of the halved aubergines and arrange them, cut-side down, on a grill pan. Place under a preheated hot grill for 7–10 minutes until charred.
....

Mix together the miso paste, two-thirds of the rice wine vinegar, the sugar and sake or water. Turn the aubergines over and brush with the miso mixture. Return to the grill for 3–5 minutes until the aubergines are soft, then sprinkle with the sesame seeds and cook for 1 minute more.
....

Meanwhile, cook the edamame beans in a saucepan of lightly salted boiling water for 2 minutes or until soft. Drain and cool under cold running water. Toss the beans in a large bowl with the rice noodles, cucumber slices, spring onions and the remaining vinegar. Season to taste and serve with the grilled miso aubergines.
....

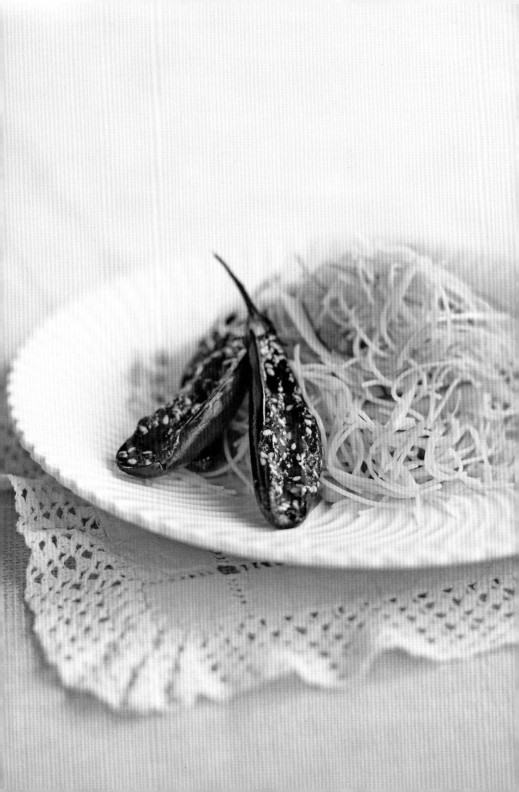

SESAME-CRUSTED TUNA WITH GINGER DRESSING

Zingy Asian flavours and omega-rich tuna: this can be served on its own or with steamed pak choi and some brown rice.

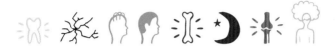

Preparation time: 15 minutes
Cooking time: 15 minutes
Serves 6

....

800 g (1 lb 10 oz) piece of fresh **tuna**
2 tbsps **vegetable oil**
3 tbsps **white sesame seeds**
3 tbsps **black sesame seeds**
½ **cucumber**, sliced into ribbons
2 **avocados**, peeled, pitted and sliced
2 **spring onions**, shredded
sea salt and **black pepper**

Dressing
1 **garlic clove**, crushed
1 **chilli**, deseeded and finely chopped
1 tsp finely chopped fresh **root ginger**
1 tbsp **light soy sauce**
juice of ½ **lime**
1 tsp finely grated **orange** rind
1 tbsp **honey**
1 tbsp **sesame oil**

Season the tuna all over. Heat the oil in a large frying pan over a high heat, add the tuna and cook for 3–5 minutes, turning from time to time, until browned all over.

Put the sesame seeds on a plate and press the seared tuna into them until well coated on all sides. Transfer the tuna to a baking sheet and place in a preheated oven, 220°C (425°F), Gas Mark 7, for 10–12 minutes until golden on the outside but still pink inside.

Mix the dressing ingredients in a small bowl. Cut the tuna into thick slices and arrange on plates with the cucumber slices, avocado pieces and spring onions. Drizzle over the dressing to serve.

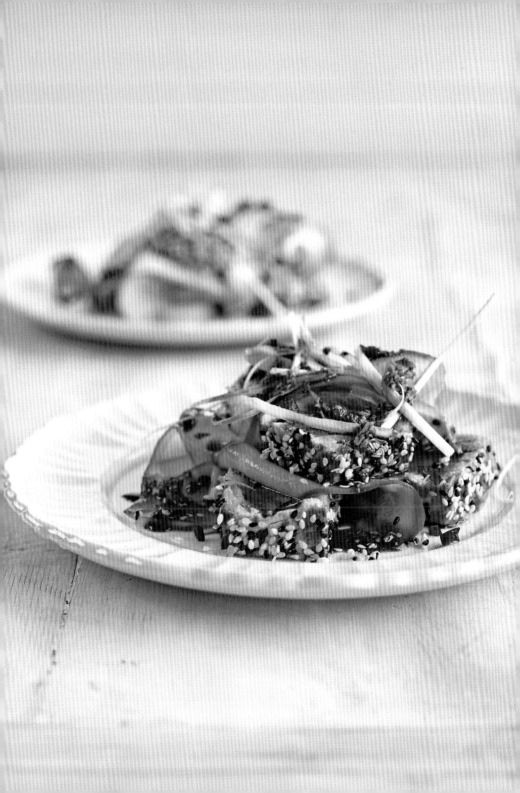

TUNA WITH PEPPERS & FENNEL GRATIN

Tuna, red peppers and fennel are key anti-ageing foods, and this tasty meal will undoubtedly become a favourite standby.

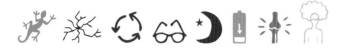

Preparation time: 20 minutes, plus cooling
Cooking time: 45 minutes
Serves 4

4 **red peppers**
6 tbsps **olive oil**
1 **garlic clove**, crushed
1 tsp **thyme** leaves
1 tsp chopped **basil**
1 tsp chopped **chives**
1 tsp **dried oregano**
4 fresh **tuna steaks**
sea salt and **black pepper**

Fennel gratin
3 large **fennel bulbs**, cut into wedges
2 **garlic cloves**, crushed
¼ tsp grated **nutmeg**
200 ml (7 fl oz) **double cream**
50 g (2 oz) **Parmesan cheese**
50 g (2 oz) **feta cheese**

Place the whole peppers under a preheated hot grill for 10–15 minutes, turning from time to time, until they are black and blistered all over. Place in a plastic bag and set aside for 15 minutes, then peel the skins off them. Remove the cores and seeds, cut the flesh into strips and place in a shallow bowl with 5 tablespoons of the olive oil, the garlic and herbs. Season to taste and set aside.

Cook the fennel wedges in a large saucepan of lightly salted water for about 5 minutes, then transfer to a shallow ovenproof dish with a slotted spoon. Add the garlic, nutmeg and cream, season to taste and mix to coat. Sprinkle over the Parmesan cheese, then crumble the feta on top. Grind over a little more pepper and cook in a preheated oven, 180°C (350°F), Gas Mark 4, for 20 minutes until golden and bubbling.

Brush the tuna steaks with the remaining oil, season to taste and place under a preheated hot grill for 2–3 minutes on each side until golden on the outside but still pink inside. Set aside to rest for a few minutes.

Arrange the marinated peppers on 4 plates, slice the tuna and lay on top. Serve with the fennel gratin.

BUTTERNUT, BROCCOLI & MUSHROOM GRATIN

Comfort food par excellence, with a boost of B vitamins and a host of antioxidants to make you look and feel younger.

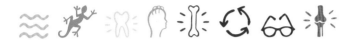

Preparation time: 15 minutes
Cooking time: 15 minutes
Serves 4
....

200 g (7 oz) **purple sprouting broccoli**, trimmed
300 g (10 oz) peeled and deseeded **butternut squash**, chopped
200 g (7 oz) **button mushrooms**, halved
60 g (2¼ oz) **butter**
2 tbsps **wholemeal flour**
400 ml (14 fl oz) **milk**
2 tsps **wholegrain mustard**
100 g (3½ oz) **Cheddar cheese**, grated
sea salt and **black pepper**

Steam the vegetables in a steamer over a saucepan of gently simmering water for 8-10 minutes until tender.
....

Meanwhile, melt the butter in a saucepan over a low heat, then stir in the wholemeal flour to make a roux. Cook for 1-2 minutes, then gradually whisk in the milk and cook, stirring continuously, until the sauce is thick and smooth. Stir in the mustard and half the grated cheese and season to taste.
....

Transfer the vegetables to an ovenproof dish, pour over the sauce and sprinkle with the remaining Cheddar cheese. Place under a preheated hot grill for 5-6 minutes until bubbling and golden. Serve immediately.
....

CARAMELIZED GARLIC TART

A nod must go in the direction of chef Yotam Ottolenghi, whose recipe inspired this dish, a big boost of anti-ageing nutrients.

Preparation time: 20 minutes
Cooking time: 55 minutes
Serves 6–8

....

400 g (13 oz) **ready-made puff pastry**
flour, for dusting
3 heads of **garlic**, cloves
separated and peeled
1 **fennel bulb**, sliced
1 tbsp **olive oil**
2 **red onions**, thinly sliced
1 tbsp **balsamic vinegar**
250 ml (8 fl oz) **water**
1 tbsp **caster sugar**
1 tsp **rosemary** leaves, chopped
1 tsp **thyme** leaves
150 g (5 oz) soft **goats' cheese**, chopped
100 g (3½ oz) **feta cheese**, chopped
50 g (2 oz) **Parmesan cheese**, grated
2 **eggs**, lightly beaten
125 ml (4 fl oz) **double cream**
90 ml (3¼ fl oz) **live Greek yogurt**
sea salt and **black pepper**

Roll out the puff pastry on a lightly floured surface to 4 mm (⅜ inch) thick and use to line a greased 30 cm (12 inch) tart tin. Cover it with nonstick baking paper and baking beans and cook blind in a pre-heated oven, 180°C (350°F), Gas Mark 4, for 20 minutes. Remove the beans and paper and cook for a further 5 minutes, until light brown.

....

Meanwhile, cook the garlic and fennel in a saucepan of boiling water for 3–4 minutes, then drain.

....

Heat the oil in a frying pan over a medium heat and add the garlic, fennel and onions. Fry for 5 minutes until the onion begins to soften. Add the vinegar and measurement water and bring to the boil. Lower the heat and simmer, uncovered, for about 10 minutes. Stir in the sugar, rosemary and thyme, season to taste, and cook, stirring frequently, until the vegetables are caramelized and the liquid has evaporated.

....

Dot the cheeses over the base of the pastry, then arrange the vegetables on top. Whisk together the eggs, cream and yogurt until light and fluffy, season to taste then pour over the cheese and vegetables. Return to the oven for 30 minutes, or until the egg mixture has set and turned golden brown.

....

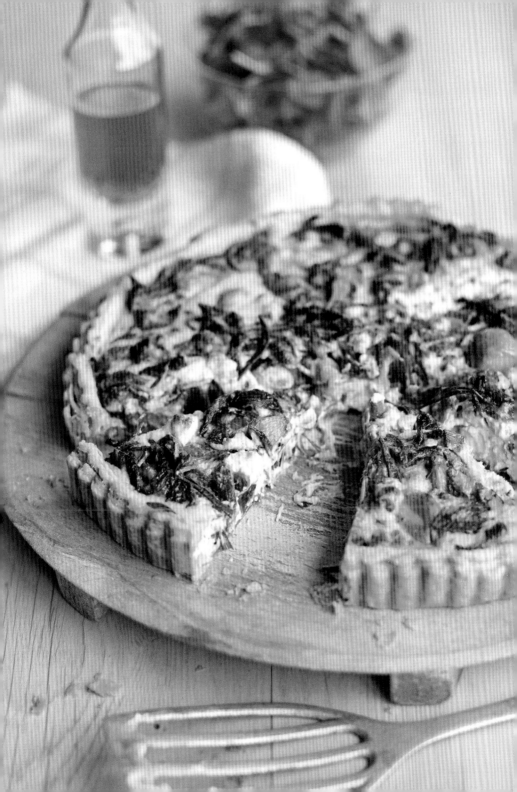

HEARTY RATATOUILLE

This one-pot meal is brimming with antioxidants and fibre to encourage overall health and wellbeing.

Preparation time: 15 minutes, plus salting
Cooking time: 1 hour–1 hour 15 minutes
Serves 4

2 large **aubergines**
2 large **courgettes**
3 tbsps **olive oil**
2 large **onions**, sliced
2 **red peppers**, cored, deseeded and cut into chunks
1 **fennel bulb**, cut into chunks
2 **garlic cloves**, crushed
400 g (13 oz) can **cherry tomatoes** in juice
1 tsp **balsamic vinegar**
1 tsp **dried oregano**
handful of **basil**, torn
sea salt and **black pepper**

Slice the aubergines and courgettes into large chunks and place them in a colander. Sprinkle with 1½ teaspoons of sea salt and toss, then transfer the chunks to a clean tea towel, wrap the towel tightly and set aside for 30 minutes to an hour.

Heat the olive oil in a large, heavy-based saucepan over a low heat and fry the onions for 5–10 minutes until just soft. Add the red peppers, fennel chunks and garlic and cook for a further 5 minutes. Then squeeze the aubergines and courgettes in the tea towel to remove excess liquid and add to the pan.

Cook for a few minutes more, then add the tomatoes, vinegar and oregano. Cover and bring to the boil, then reduce the heat and simmer for 45 minutes or until the tomatoes have broken down and the vegetables have become tender.

Stir in half the basil and season to taste if necessary. Cook, uncovered, for a further 10–15 minutes, until the sauce thickens. Serve scattered with the remaining basil.

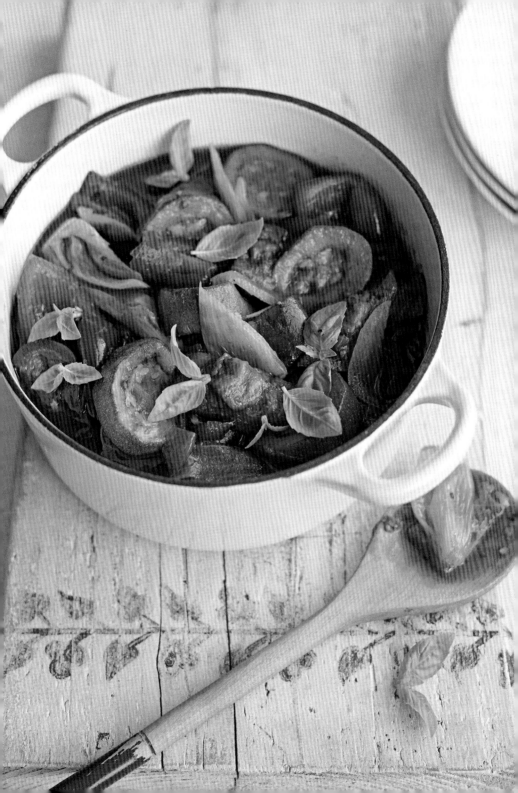

AUBERGINE, CHICKPEA & PANEER CURRY

This robust curry is quick and easy to make, and full of nutrients to reduce the impact of ageing on all parts of your body.

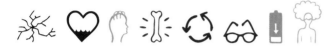

Preparation time: 20 minutes, plus salting
Cooking time: 45 minutes–1 hour
Serves 4

1 large **aubergine**
1 tbsp **olive oil**
2 **garlic cloves**, crushed
2 **onions**, chopped
7.5 cm (3 inch) piece of fresh **root ginger**, grated, plus extra to serve
1 tsp mild **chilli powder**
1 tsp **ground cumin**
½ tsp **garam masala**, plus extra to serve
½ tsp **ground coriander**
½ tsp **ground turmeric**
2 x 400 g (13 oz) cans **chickpeas**, rinsed and drained
400 ml (13 fl oz) **coconut milk**
60 ml (2½ fl oz) **live natural yogurt**
handful of **mint** leaves, chopped
200 g (7 oz) **paneer cheese**, cubed
75 g (3 oz) fresh **coriander**, chopped
sea salt and **black pepper**

Chop the aubergine into chunks and place in a colander. Sprinkle with 1½ teaspoons of sea salt and toss, then transfer the chunks to a clean tea towel, wrap the towel tightly and set aside for 30 minutes to an hour.
....

Heat the oil in a large saucepan or wok over a low heat and add the garlic, onions and ginger. Cook for about 10 minutes, stirring often, until the onions are soft and starting to caramelize. Squeeze the aubergines in the tea towel to remove excess liquid then add to the pan.
....

Add the chilli powder, cumin, garam masala, ground coriander and turmeric and cook for a further 2–3 minutes. Add the chickpeas and coconut milk, stir well, cover and simmer for 20–30 minutes. Remove the lid and cook for a further 10 minutes, mashing some of the chickpeas into the sauce to thicken.
....

Meanwhile, mix the yogurt in a bowl with the mint, season to taste and set aside. Heat a nonstick frying pan over a medium heat, add the paneer and cook briefly, stirring, until golden all over. Tip the cheese into the curry, season if necessary and add a pinch of garam masala, a grating of fresh ginger and the fresh coriander and toss to mix. Serve with the minty yogurt on the side.
....

SPAGHETTI WITH OLIVE OIL, GARLIC & CHILLI

The simplicity of this dish belies the huge range of nutrients it contains. It's particularly good for skin, hair and joints.

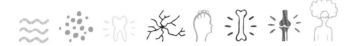

Preparation time: 5 minutes
Cooking time: 10-15 minutes
Serves 4
....

400 g (13 oz) **wholewheat spaghetti**
8 tbsps **olive oil**
4 **garlic cloves**, finely chopped
2 small **red chillies**, deseeded
and finely chopped
sea salt and **black pepper**
handful of **parsley**, chopped, to garnish
grated **pecorino cheese**, to serve (optional)

Cook the spaghetti in a large saucepan of lightly salted water according to packet instructions until al dente.
....

Heat the oil in a large, heavy-based frying pan over a low heat and add the garlic and chilli. Cook gently for 1-2 minutes until the garlic just starts to turn golden.
....

Drain the pasta and transfer it to the frying pan with a few tablespoons of the cooking water. Season to taste and toss to coat the pasta in the oil. Transfer to a dish, scatter with parsley and serve with the pecorino, if liked.
....

BAKED HONEY, CARDAMOM & CINNAMON FIGS

Cinnamon is known for its beneficial effect on joints, but did you know it also aids digestion, circulation and bone health?

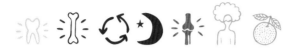

Preparation time: 5 minutes
Cooking time: 25 minutes
Serves 4

12 ripe **figs**
1 tbsp **ghee** or **butter**, plus extra for greasing
2 tsps **cardamom seeds**
2 **cinnamon sticks**
finely grated rind of 1 **lemon**
4–5 tbsps **honey**
icing sugar, for dusting
live Greek yogurt, to serve

Cut a deep cross down through the stalk end of each fig, keeping the base intact, and put in a lightly greased ovenproof dish.

Melt the ghee or butter in a small saucepan, stir in the cardamom seeds, cinnamon sticks, grated lemon rind and honey and cook for 2 minutes until bubbling. Pour the mixture evenly over the figs.

Place in a preheated oven, 200°C (400°F), Gas Mark 6, for 20 minutes until sizzling. Dust with icing sugar and serve with yogurt.

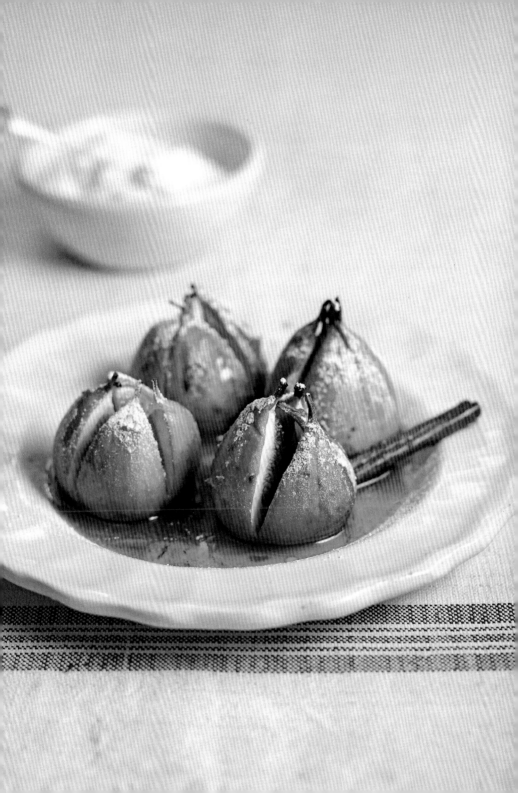

FRUIT SALSA & CINNAMON CRISPS

This delicious, light dessert is full of antioxidants to boost the health and wellbeing of the whole family.

Preparation time: 15 minutes, plus cooling
Cooking time: 10 minutes
Serves 4

1 **kiwi fruit**, peeled and diced
100 g (3½ oz) **blackberries**, halved
100 g (3½ oz) **strawberries**, hulled and sliced
100 g (3½ oz) **raspberries**, halved
1 **Pink Lady apple**, cored and diced
1 **pear**, cored and diced
50 g (2 oz) **pomegranate seeds**
1 tbsp **pomegranate molasses**
finely grated rind and juice of 1 **orange**
1 tsp **ground cinnamon**
½ tsp **ground ginger**
2 tbsps **honey**
3 tbsps chopped **mint**

Cinnamon crips
1 tbsp **olive oil**
1 tsp **ground cinnamon**
1 tbsp **honey**
2 soft **wholewheat tortillas**

Mix all the salsa ingredients in a large bowl, cover and set aside for the flavours to blend.

For the cinnamon crisps, whisk the olive oil, cinnamon and honey together and brush over both sides of the tortillas. Use a sharp knife or pizza wheel to cut the tortillas into triangles, then arrange on a baking sheet and put in a preheated oven, 180°C (350°F), Gas Mark 4, for 10 minutes or until just crisp. Allow to cool.

Serve the fruit salsa in a big dipping dish or in individual ramekins, with the tortillas on the side. Any leftover salsa can be kept in an airtight container in the refrigerator for up to 4 days.

CHOCOLATE PUDDLE PUDDINGS

A sumptuous dark chocolate dessert which will improve your mood, while also helping your skin, teeth, hair, heart and brain.

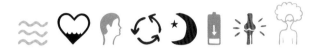

Preparation time: 10 minutes
Cooking time: 25 minutes
Serves 2
....

75 g (3 oz) **butter**, plus extra for greasing
75 g (3 oz) **golden caster sugar**
75 g (3 oz) **dark chocolate**,
broken into pieces
2 small **eggs**
25 g (1 oz) **plain flour**

To serve
cream
blackberries

Grease 2 individual ovenproof ramekins or pudding basins and sprinkle with 1 teaspoon of the sugar.
....

Place the chocolate and butter in a heatproof bowl set over a saucepan of simmering water and stir gently until melted and smooth.
....

Whisk the eggs and the remaining sugar with a hand-held electric whisk until very thick, pale and creamy. Whisk in the melted chocolate mixture, then lightly fold in the flour.
....

Spoon the mixture into the prepared basins or ramekins and place on a baking sheet. Place in a preheated oven, 190°C (375°F), Gas Mark 5, for 15–20 minutes until firm on the outside but still wobbly in the centre.
....

Turn the puddings out into 2 bowls and serve warm with cream and blackberries.
....

BANANAS WITH SPICED CHOCOLATE

The resveratrol in dark chocolate, the polyphenols in cinnamon and the B vitamins in bananas put the anti-ageing proof in this decadent pudding.

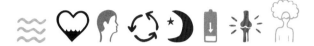

Preparation time: 5 minutes
Cooking time: 5 minutes
Serves 4

200 g (7 oz) **dark chocolate**,
broken into pieces
25 g (1 oz) **unsalted butter**
1 tbsp **honey**
1 piece of **stem ginger in syrup**,
drained and finely diced
1 tsp **ground cinnamon**
4 ripe **bananas**, sliced

To serve
2 tbsps **flaked almonds**, toasted
live natural yogurt (optional)

Place the chocolate, butter, honey, ginger and cinnamon in a heatproof bowl set over a saucepan of simmering water and stir gently until the chocolate has melted.

Divide the sliced bananas between 4 bowls. Pour over the chocolate sauce and serve sprinkled with the almonds and some live yogurt, if liked.

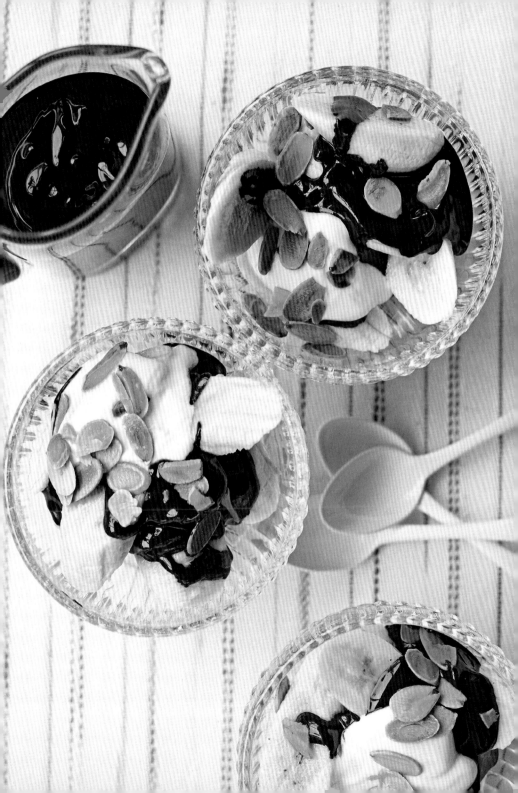

CRANBERRY ICE CREAM WITH DARK CHOCOLATE

This mouthwatering dessert is packed with of antioxidants, calcium and a whole host of nutrients to rejuvenate and uplift.

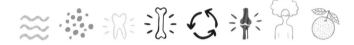

Preparation time: 10 minutes, plus cooling and freezing
Cooking time: 15 minutes
Serves 6
....

400 g (13 oz) **cranberries**
90 ml (3¼ fl oz) **water**
1 tsp **ground cinnamon**
150 g (5 oz) **golden caster sugar**
seeds scraped from 1 **vanilla pod**
600 ml (1 pint) **whipping cream**
200 ml (7 fl oz) **live natural yogurt**
50 g (2 oz) **dark chocolate chips**

Place the cranberries, measurement water, cinnamon and one-third of the sugar in a saucepan over a medium heat. Bring to the boil, reduce the heat, cover and cook for about 10 minutes, or until the cranberries have softened into the liquid. Allow to cool for 20 minutes, mashing the fruit with a fork.
....

Place the mixture in a food processor and pulse until roughly chopped.
....

Place the remaining sugar, the vanilla seeds, whipping cream and live yogurt in a heavy-based saucepan over a medium heat and stir until the sugar has dissolved, then stir in the cranberry mixture.
....

Transfer to a shallow dish and place in the freezer for about 1 hour. Stir in the chocolate chips and freeze again for a further hour, or until softly set.
....

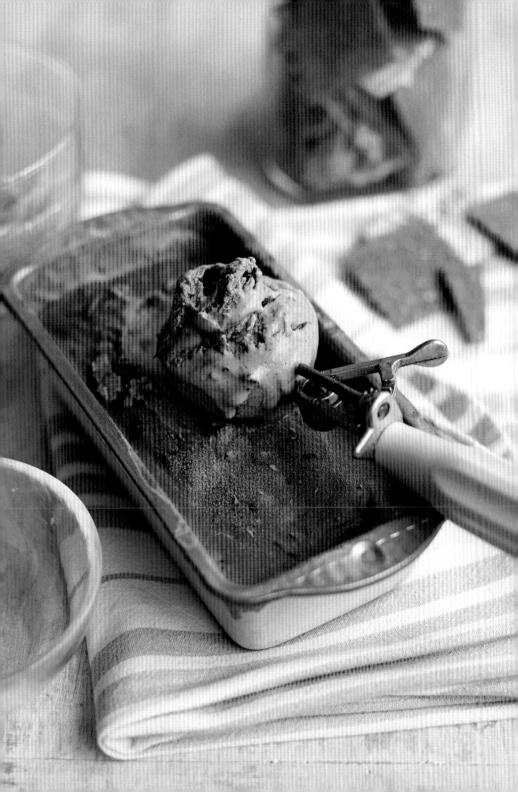

GUAVA ICE CREAM WITH BLACKBERRY COULIS

This is an easy recipe that can be prepared in advance to supply a burst of fibre, antioxidants and vitamins to turn back the clock.

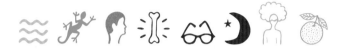

Preparation time: 10 minutes, plus freezing
Cooking time: 20 minutes
Serves 4-6

6 ripe **guavas**, peeled, deseeded and diced
100 g (3½oz) **golden granulated sugar**
finely grated rind and juice of 1 **lime**
600 ml (1 pint) **whipping cream**
1 tsp **vanilla extract**

Coulis
200 g (7 oz) **blackberries**
2 tbsps **honey**
60 ml (2½ fl oz) **water**

Place the diced guava, sugar, and lime rind and juice in a shallow dish and place in the freezer for about 2 hours, or until just frozen.

Meanwhile, place the blackberries, honey and measurement water in a small, heavy-based saucepan over a medium heat. Bring to the boil then reduce the heat and simmer, mashing the blackberries into the liquid from time to time, for 15 minutes or until thick. The purée can be strained through a sieve if you like, but the seeds are also rich in nutrients. Set aside to cool.

Whisk the cream and vanilla extract in a food processor until it forms soft peaks, then add the guava mixture and blitz until smooth. Serve immediately with the coulis, or store in the freezer until ready to serve.

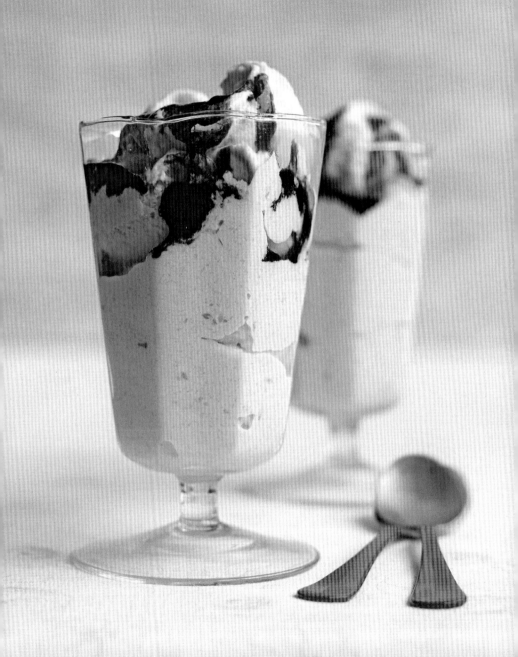

POMEGRANATE PANNA COTTA

This super-easy-to-make dessert is rich in calcium and anti-ageing antioxidants to keep your bones strong and your skin, hair and mood glowing.

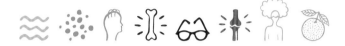

Preparation time: 10 minutes, plus chilling
Cooking time: 5 minutes
Serves 6

4 leaves of **gelatine**
1 **vanilla pod**, split lengthways
600 ml (1 pint) **double cream**
200 ml (7 fl oz) **semi-skimmed milk**
175 g (6 oz) **golden caster sugar**
50 g (2 oz) **pomegranate seeds**,
plus extra to decorate
finely grated rind of ½ **orange**
2 tbsps **pomegranate molasses**
2 tbsps **orange juice**
mint leaves, to decorate

Soak the gelatine in a cup of cold water for about 5 minutes until softened.

Scrape the seeds out of the vanilla pod and place in a large, heavy-based saucepan with the pod, the cream, milk and sugar. Bring to the boil over a medium heat, stirring continuously until the sugar has dissolved. Remove from the heat and remove the vanilla pod.

Squeeze the gelatine leaves to remove any excess water, then add to the pan one by one and stir until dissolved.

Wet the insides of 6 large ramekins with cold water and set aside. Mix together the pomegranate seeds and orange rind in a small bowl and spoon the mixture into the bases of the ramekins. Pour in the vanilla cream and chill in the refrigerator for 2–3 hours until set.

To serve, dip the ramekins in hot water for a few seconds, then turn out the panna cottas on to serving plates. Whisk the pomegranate molasses with the orange juice and drizzle over the top. Sprinkle the panna cottas with a few extra pomegranate seeds and mint leaves to decorate.

BLACKBERRY BRÛLÉES

These divine pots, with all the nutrient power of shiny purple blackberries, are quick to prepare and slip down a treat.

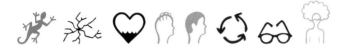

Preparation time: 5 minutes, plus cooling
Cooking time: 5 minutes
Serves 4
....

225 g (7½ oz) **blackberries**
2 tbsps pressed **apple juice**
2–3 tsps **caster sugar**
8 tbsps **live Greek yogurt**
2 tbsps soft dark **brown sugar**

Place the blackberries, apple juice and caster sugar, to taste, in a saucepan over a medium heat, bring to the boil then reduce the heat and simmer for 2–3 minutes. Spoon into 4 ramekins and leave to cool for 2–3 minutes.
....

Spoon over the yogurt, then sprinkle with the brown sugar. Cover and chill until required.
....

APPLE & BLACKBERRY COMPOTE WITH ALMOND SCONES

A lovely autumnal dish with all the antioxidant goodness of apples and blackberries, and vitamin E from the almonds.

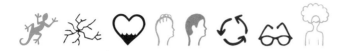

Preparation time: 20 minutes
Cooking time: 15 minutes
Serves 4
....

400 g (13 oz) **Bramley apples**, peeled, cored and sliced
2 tbsps **water**
150 g (5 oz) **blackberries**
2 tbsps **apricot jam**
live vanilla-flavoured Greek yogurt, to serve

Scones
125 g (4 oz) **self-raising flour**, plus extra for dusting
50 g (2 oz) **ground almonds**
75 g (3 oz) **caster sugar**
50 g (2 oz) **butter**
6 tbsps **milk**, plus extra for brushing
1 tsp **vanilla extract**
25 g (1 oz) **flaked almonds**

To make the scones, place the flour, ground almonds, caster sugar and butter in a food processor and pulse until the mixture forms fine crumbs. Add the milk and vanilla extract and pulse again to make a soft dough. Turn out the dough on to a lightly floured surface and knead briefly. Press it out using your fingers, then stamp out 8 rounds using a 7 cm (3 inch) cutter.

Place the scones on a floured baking sheet, brush with a little milk and sprinkle with the flaked almonds. Then place in a preheated oven, 200°C (400°F), Gas Mark 6, for about 10–15 minutes until golden.

Meanwhile, place the apples in a saucepan with the measurement water and cook for 3 minutes until soft. Stir in the blackberries and apricot jam and simmer for 1 minute.

Spoon the compote into 4 bowls and serve warm or cold with the scones and yogurt.

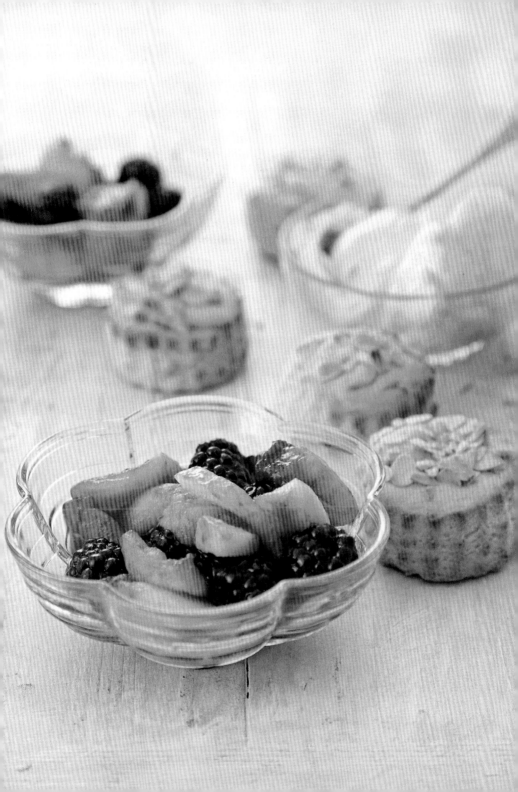

RESOURCES

Action on Addiction
Tel: 0300 330 0659
Email: action@actiononaddiction.org.uk
Website: www.actiononaddiction.org.uk

Age UK
Helpline: 0800 169 6565
Website: www.ageuk.org.uk

Anxiety UK
Tel: 0161 227 9898
Email: info@anxietyuk.org.uk
Website: www.anxietyuk.org.uk

Arthritis Research UK (joint health)
Tel: 0300 790 0400
Website: www.arthritisresearchuk.org

British Dental Health Foundation
Helpline: 0845 063 1188
Website: www.dentalhealth.org

British Heart Foundation
Helpline: 020 7935 0185
Website: www.bhf.org.uk

British Meditation Society
Tel: 01460 62921
Website: www.britishmeditationsociety.org

British Nutrition Foundation
Tel: 020 7557 7930
Email: postbox@nutrition.org.uk
Website: www.nutrition.org.uk

British Wheel of Yoga
Tel: 01529 306 851
Website: www.bwy.org.uk

Diabetes UK
Tel: 0845 120 2960
Email: info@diabetes.org.uk
Website: www.diabetes.org.uk

The Eyecare Trust
Tel: 0845 129 5001
Email: info@eyecaretrust.org.uk
Website: www.eyecaretrust.org.uk

Institute for Food, Brain and Behaviour
Tel: 0800 644 0322
Website: www.ifbb.org.uk

National Osteoporosis Society
Helpline: 0845 450 0230
Website: www.nos.org.uk

The Nutrition Society
Tel: 020 7602 0228
Email: office@nutritionsociety.org
Website: www.nutritionsociety.org

Pain Concern
Tel: 0300 123 0789
Email: info@painconcern.org.uk
Website: www.painconcern.org.uk

Patient.co.uk (relaxation exercises)
Website: www.patient.co.uk/health/relaxation-exercises

Sleep Matters Insomnia Helpline
Tel: 020 8994 9874 (6pm to 8pm)

Stress Management Society
Tel: 08701 999 235
Email: info@stress.org.uk
Website: www.stress.org.uk

INDEX

ACKNOWLEDGEMENTS

Thinkstock Alexander Kovalchuk 20; Frans Rombout 7; gemenacom 30; Hemera Technologies 12; Jovan Nikolic 8; Natikka 17; pattymalajak 9; sommail 28; Wavebreakmedia Ltd 27.